Mental Health
Services in Disasters:
Instructor's Guide

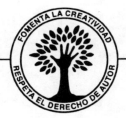

EL LIBRO MUERE CUANDO LO FOTOCOPIA

AMIGO LECTOR:

La obra que usted tiene en sus manos posee un gran valor.
En ella, su autor ha vertido conocimientos, experiencia y mucho trabajo. El editor ha procurado una presentación digna de su contenido y está poniendo todo su empeño y recursos para que sea ampliamente difundida, a través de su red de comercialización.

Al fotocopiar este libro, el autor y el editor dejan de percibir lo que corresponde a la inversión que ha realizado y se desalienta la creación de nuevas obras. Rechace cualquier ejemplar «pirata» o fotocopia ilegal de este libro, pues de lo contrario estará contribuyendo al lucro de quienes se aprovechan ilegítimamente del esfuerzo del autor y del editor.

La reproducción no autorizada de obras protegidas por el derecho de autor no sólo es un delito, sino que atenta contra la creatividad y la difusión de la cultura.

Para mayor información comuníquese con nosotros:

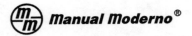

Editorial El Manual Moderno, S.A. de C.V.
Av. Sonora 206, Col. Hipódromo, 06100
México, D.F.

Editorial El Manual Moderno (Colombia), Ltda
Carrera 12-A No. 79-03/05
Santafé de Bogotá

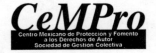

Mental Health Services in Disasters:

Instructor's Guide

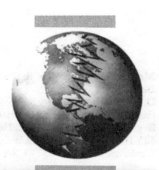

RAQUEL E. COHEN, M.D., M.P.H.
University of Miami School of Medicine
Miami, Florida

Pan American Health Organization

Editorial El Manual Moderno
México, D.F. – Santafé de Bogotá

Mental Health Services in Disasters:
Instructor's Guide
D.R. Copyright 2000 by the:
Pan American Health Organization (PAHO/WHO)
Regional Office of the World Health Organization
525 Twenty-third Street, N.W.
Washington, D.C. 20037 - USA

ISBN 92-75-12274-1 (Pan American Health Organization)

Published also in Spanish with the title:
Salud Mental para Víctimas de Desastres:
Guía para instructores

A publication of the Emergency Preparedness and Disaster Relief
Coordination Program, PAHO/WHO.

The production of this publication has been made possible through
the financial support of the International Humanitarian Assistance
Division of the Canadian International Development Agency
(IHA/CIDA), the Office of Foreign Disaster Assistance of the U.S.
Agency for International Development (OFDA/AID), and the
Department for International Development of the U.K (DFID).

In co-edition with:
Editorial El Manual Moderno, S.A. de C.V.,
Av. Sonora núm. 206,
Col. Hipódromo,
Deleg. Cuauhtémoc
06100 México, D.F.

ISBN 968-426-879-3 (Editorial El Manual Moderno)

Member of the National Chamber of the Mexican Editorial
Industry, Reg. No. 39

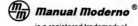

Pan American Health Organization

"When the center of someone's life has been blown out like the core of a building, is it any wonder if it takes so long even to find a door to close?"

Ellen Goodman
The Boston Globe
January 4, 1998

Glossary*

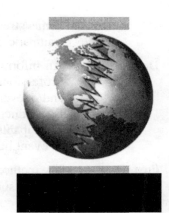

Disaster survivor

Any individual or family who should be offered assistance after a disaster.

Coping behaviors/ oping strategies

The ways in which an individual addresses or responds to a stressful incident. These ways can be adaptive and contribute to decreased stress, or they can be maladaptive and fail to decrease stress and/or cause secondary problems.

Outreach

Providing emotional support during the acute period following a disaster. Outreach is designed to assist survivors in expressing and understanding disaster-caused stress and grief reactions, and aid a return to a state of equilibrium.

Debriefing

A formal session, led by a specially trained mental health professional, usually within a few days of a critical incident and/or at the end of an assignment involving one or more intense stressors. A debriefing provides an opportunity for participants to express and share their feeling with others exposed to the

---

* Adapted from American Red Cross. *Disaster Mental Health Provider's Course.* Washington, D.C.: American Red Cross; 1991. (ARC 3076A).

same stressors, to learn about typical human reactions to traumatic experiences, and to discuss adaptive coping strategies.

Defusing

An informal session, led by a specially trained mental health professional, usually within a few days of a critical incident and/or event involving one or more intense stressors. A defusing is conducted in an atmosphere of mutual support, with the participants describing their feelings and reactions to the incident or event being discussed.

Post-disaster intervention

The method accepted by counselors for addressing mental health needs of survivors. Any treatment or assistance outside the scope of crisis counseling should be referred to other agencies.

Intrapshychic issues

Unresolved psychological issues, personality traits, or patterns of defending against anxiety that are within or intrinsic to an individual and that contribute to the ways in which the individual responds to a traumatic event.

Mental health emergency

An emotional or behavioral response that is beyond the scope of crisis counseling services and therefore requires mental health intervention provided through more comprehensive resources. Emergencies include, but are not limited to, responses demonstrating a threat to the safety of an individual or others, substance abuse, seriously impaired functioning, and significant symptoms that persist despite crisis counseling interventions.

Contents

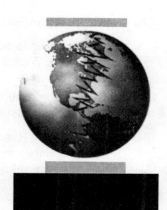

Introduction

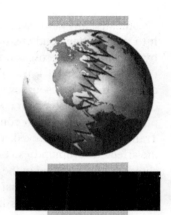

◼◼ HOW TO USE THIS TRAINING GUIDE

◼ KEY ISSUES IN TRAINING

This training guide is designed as an accompanying volume to *Disaster Mental Health Services: Manual for Workers*. It will help in the training and supervision of individuals who assist survivors to respond effectively to the aftermath of disasters. For the purposes of this guide, mental health workers will be identified as post-disaster counselors or workers, in contrast to all other agency emergency workers. These workers may come from a variety of disciplines and levels, ranging from degreed professionals to paraprofessionals. The mix and match within the teams assembled after a disaster will vary according to the region of the world in which the disaster occurs and the human resources available. The trainers will be individuals who are prepared to teach multidisciplinary teams of workers. They, in turn, will collaborate with other workers from different agencies—including mental health clinics, the Red Cross, alcohol and drug abuse agencies, churches, and the civil defense—in the event that they require additional resources or need to refer survivors for further treatment.

Ideally, this guide will be used as an aid for trainers who can translate and adapt it to the language and customs of a region before a disaster, but it can also be used by mental health professionals who need to prepare a post-disaster team to move rapidly to the front lines. The trainers who are hired to train disaster teams may develop training resources in addition to those presented in the pages of this guide, or they may develop their own versions of the exercises, scripts or vignettes for role-playing. They may also contribute personal experiences from their own countries. Trainers might also be asked to provide post-disaster education and consultation to the affected communities. To perform these activities successfully, these individuals should be well trained in the various techniques before a disaster. Alternatively, they might recruit experts to assist them in presenting certain contents.

The objective for this kind of generic training for post-disaster workers is to have a well-prepared and skilled group of workers who can respond effectively in the aftermath of a disaster and participate in post-disaster mental health programs that have been designed, organized, and administratively developed for the people in the community in which they live. To attain this objective, training should be planned before a disaster occurs so that services are offered by workers who have been trained to enter the disaster area with a clear knowledge of their responsibilities. It is also important to incorporate and develop appropriate mechanisms to build effective liaisons with the emergency agencies participating in the community effort as part of the training in mental health for post-disaster programs in the country.

This preparation for disaster response requires that a training program be conducted for the workers of the mental health agencies that will deliver post-disaster counseling programs—encompassing education, consultation, outreach, crisis intervention, and mental health supportive services. Providing this training means acquiring information on the needs of the affected community and the consequences of the disorganization of human services. Such information is often lacking, inadequate, or unreliable, especially in the first few weeks after disaster strikes. As a result, decisions to deploy services are based on assumptions, which makes it essential to continually reevaluate and redefine program support as part of ongoing training. A fundamental principle of training for disaster mental health workers is to adapt the basic, generic contents to the specific characteristics of the region's official emergency response and to provide continuous training throughout all the phases of the post-disaster period.

DEFINITION OF TRAINING

"Training" means the specific instruction which may be required to enable disaster workers to provide crisis counseling to a survivor of a major disaster or its aftermath (in contrast to instruction for clinical procedures). Training also means the instruction that may be required for all other caregivers, professionals, public agency emergency workers, and mental health specialists in disaster assistance programs so that they will be more sensitive to possible mental health problems of survivors and will know when to refer such survivors to the mental health agencies serving the disaster programs.

Trainers are responsible for organizing and conducting training courses for the groups that will deliver assistance to agencies and survivors recovering from the impact of a natural disaster.

This manual for the training of post-disaster teams for post-disaster intervention programs has been developed in response to the need to produce trained workers who can be mobilized after a disaster. The trainers will organize and conduct training for participants for whom post-disaster intervention is a secondary and novel job and who will have limited time to prepare themselves.

The organization of the material in this training guide assumes that the trainers already possess the skills, knowledge, and attitudes needed to teach the post-disaster crisis counselors.

For training in post-disaster intervention to be effective, the experienced professional who will serve as a trainer needs to have competence in the training approaches that have been successfully developed to train adults. Trainers must be able not only to train persons in post-disaster intervention methodology, but also to devise training strategies that help ensure that relevant approaches are selected for the program mandated by the agencies. The target groups and types of training that workers will need will depend on the particular context of a post-disaster situation and the responsibilities of the workers.

Trainers should be able to organize and conduct training courses for different groups, which may vary in composition, background, ethnicity, and level of preparation. This is one of the challenges of training post-disaster teams: their variability poses an educational challenge for organizing the methods and content in such a way as to meet the training needs of every member of the team. Not only does the material need to be relevant and make sense to the worker, but it needs to be operationally driven in order to help individuals traumatized by the disaster. Although the content of training will vary for different groups, the basic training methods and the issues that should be considered in organizing and conducting training courses for all groups are similar, though they will need to be adapted to the circumstances surrounding the event, the characteristics of the population, and the amount of damage and disorganization in the community. For these reasons, the training guide and the manual for workers include basic content which leaves room for variation, creativity, and new possibilities in the number of resources, exercises, vignettes, and discussions. The training guide includes varying levels of content, allowing trainers to pick and choose according to the background, disciplines, and prior knowledge of their "students."

■ GOALS OF TRAINING

Continuous training is a systematic transmission of information and new knowledge to keep the individual updated on approaches, methodology, and application of existing knowledge in order to operationalize a post-disaster program when needed. The aim of such a program is to assist individuals affected by the consequences of a disaster, which may include the rupture and fragmentation of community structures, shelter, life support systems, employment, etc. Training has a role in enhancing the efficiency and effectiveness of the emergency disaster assistance program as an integral part of the overall process of community recovery.

The goal of disaster training is to prepare personnel at all levels, providing them with relevant information to enable them to solve the problems they will face. One of the defining characteristics of such work is its participatory, multiagency, multidisciplinary nature. Clearly, the involvement of multiple groups—the community, governmental and non-governmental agencies, and decision-makers—in defining needs helps focus the various types of mental health assistance and enhance the quality of services. In addition, the participation of these groups together in all stages of the effort, including crisis survivor counseling, is valuable if acceptable solutions to problems are to be implemented and sustained throughout the impacted area.

Because disaster assistance addresses mental health problems in the broad context of social, economic, and community development, inputs from many different disciplines are required. These include community demographics, social systems, behavioral sciences, governmental disaster policy and management, and clinical medicine and psychology. Each of these disciplines has developed specialized approaches in its efforts to provide information that will support post-disaster intervention programs. It is increasingly evident that the problems that have to be addressed require combined input from many disciplines and that disaster workers need to acquire the skills to work together in multidisciplinary teams.

The main characteristics of post-disaster intervention are:

• Its focus on priority problems of survivors;
• Its interactive, participatory nature;
• Its action orientation;
• Its emphasis on the here and now;
• Its focus on practical, timely solutions.

Although the methodologies of post-disaster assistance can be applied to different regions of a country, the procedures and approaches to the problems will not be the same because differences in cultural, social, economic, and political realities have an important influence on post-disaster programs. In each country, the mental health component of disaster management programs will be integrated into overall government planning. This broad area of planning, organizing, and delivering services, which links federal, state/provincial, and local efforts, is not discussed in this manual. This choice was made to add flexibility to the manual, so that it can used within the differing structures of disaster programs in various countries. Moreover, the design and organization of the disaster response structure continues to evolve in the United States, and it may differ from that in other countries. In spite of the variation in organizational structures worldwide, human reactions to trauma have been found to be very similar, which makes it possible to devise a basic approach to alleviating the suffering of survivors of many types of trauma, provided the worker is trained to recognize the different cultural components of reactions to various types of stressors and their consequences. The development of a manual to train workers in post-disaster crisis intervention responds to a clear need and addresses the reality that it is neither practical nor feasible to form an active, up-to-date professional force to react to random, occasional disasters in some part of a country. However, it is feasible to have a cadre of trainers who, with the assistance of this manual, can prepare workers, who, in turn, will become members of teams dispatched to work in affected areas.

■ DEFINITION OF POST-DISASTER MENTAL HEALTH INTERVENTION

Crisis counseling intervention to mitigate post-traumatic responses of survivors following a disaster is designed as a service of planned procedures that assist the dynamic process of the survivors' coping and adapting to the new setting by improving their ability to deal with the many problems arising after a disaster.

There is an opportunity to help survivors by focusing on their psychological coping mechanisms. Through methods that complement the more traditional somatic interventions and the functions of the professionals to whom the crisis counselor may refer for further treatment, the counselor has the opportunity to prevent future psychopathological sequelae. Crisis intervention in post-disaster programs can add a new dimension to the services provided by emergency agencies. Mental health personnel can enhance the emergency program for the population of survivors. They can provide a crisis approach that is appropriate for every at-risk survivor in a post-disaster setting. Such crisis programs seek to help survivors relearn their coping methods in the setting in which they find themselves and diminish the potential for dysfunction and pathological outcomes. The training encourages the counselor to develop a systematic approach to strengthen survivors' coping methods. For the disaster personnel, this approach can lead to: (1) increased understanding of normal stress responses in a disaster, (2) growth of esteem for the survivors, (3) development of coping and communication skills, (4) improved ability to master problem situations, and (5) development of problem-solving skills. All of these skills help improve survivors' capability to move through the process of loss and mourning in a world destroyed by disaster.

■ DEFINITION OF TERMS

Crisis intervention is a counseling method using techniques that help survivors:

1. Strengthen coping methodologies;
2. Acquire more knowledge of what is happening;

3. Explore available attitudinal and behavioral alternatives through the phases of the disaster;

4. Get through the transition processes created by the disaster and come to a satisfactory resolution of their problems.

The worker's intervention is aimed at:

1. Helping the survivor to understand and anticipate further stress;
2. Minimizing the impact of the trauma;
3. Developing and improving communication skills;
4. Strengthening problem-solving skills;
5. Improving social coping and functioning within the rapidly changing agency system in the post-disaster environment;
6. Supporting relationships both with other survivors and with agency staff;
7. Fostering coping skills and adaptation to the changes in the community that will happen after the disaster.

The following are key variables in post-disaster intervention that workers should know:

1. Identification of the problem situation;
2. Timeframe of intervention through outreach methods;
3. Screening for access to services needed by survivors;
4. Method used to assist survivors;
5. Role of the crisis counselor;
6. Supporting theories and hypotheses that will guide the intervention (crisis, loss and mourning, stressor and stress response, coping);
7. Methods of education, prevention, counseling, and referral;
8. Approach—identification of crisis responses used by the survivor and development of appropriate coping plans;
9. Emphasis on cognitive and social communication skills;
10. Orientation—focus on the "here and now" and on current interactions and dynamics, recent events, and prevention;
11. Goals for assisting survivors by increasing knowledge, developing skills and attitudes to support survivors in dealing with the crisis in their lives after the disaster;
12. Identification of behavior that is maladaptive for coping.

■ DEFINITION OF A DISASTER SURVIVOR

The term "survivor" in this manual refers to those individuals and families who have suffered from a disaster and its consequences. Disaster survivors have experienced an unexpected and stressful event. The term denotes the capacity of the individual who has been victimized by the disaster but is gathering strength and increasing his/her capacity to cope as time goes by. Perhaps most survivors were functioning adequately before the catastrophe, but their ability to cope may have been impaired by the stress of the situation. Even though the survivors may exhibit symptoms of physical or psychological stress, they <u>do</u> <u>not</u> view themselves, nor should they be viewed, as experiencing psychopathology. They are reacting in a normal way to an abnormal situation. Disaster survivors may include persons of all ages, socioeconomic classes, and race or ethnicity because catastrophes affect the entire population in an impacted area. It is assumed that individuals can resume their usual functions if aided and given emotional support and appropriate information and guidance.

Some survivors may suffer more than others, depending on several interrelated factors. Those who may be particularly susceptible to prolonged physical and psychological reactions from a disaster include people who:

• are vulnerable due to previous traumatic life events;
• are at risk due to recent ill health or chronic conditions (heart disease, HIV infection);
• experience severe prolonged stress and catastrophic loss due to the disaster;
• lose their sources of social and psychological support;
• lack coping skills.

The elderly are a group that in general may find it difficult to cope with disasters and their consequences. It is not unusual to find older survivors who are isolated from their support systems and who live alone. As a result, they are often afraid to seek help. Typical post-catastrophe outcomes in this group are depression and a sense of hopelessness. Unfortunately, a common response among some older people is a lack of interest in rebuilding their lives.

Children are also a special group because they usually do not have the capacity to understand and rationalize what has happened. Consequently, they may experience emotional or behavioral problems at home or school. Perhaps the most prominent disturbances reported in children after a disaster are phobias, sleep disturbances, loss of interest in school, and difficult behavior.

Some individuals with a history of mental illness may also require special attention. Under the stress of a disaster situation, relapses can occur in this population due to the loss of support systems or inability to obtain their daily medication.

Finally, another at-risk group to be considered by the worker are individuals experiencing certain life crises. Members of this group might include, for example, recently widowed or divorced people or those who, at the time of the disaster, had recently lost their jobs or undergone major surgery. These survivors may display a special vulnerability to the stress generated by a natural disaster.

In summary, although specific at-risk groups merit close attention from the disaster worker, everyone can be considered a survivor in a disaster area and should be offered assistance.

ORGANIZATION OF THE TRAINING MODULE CHAPTERS

The subject matter of the training program presented in this guide is distributed in five modules. Each of the five modules includes:

- Learning objectives;
- Suggestions concerning educational methods to be used in presenting the module;
- A summary of the content of the workers' manual;
- Teaching aids (transparencies or slides and handouts);
- Guidelines for group work or exercises;
- A selected list of reading materials (which may be supplemented with more up-to-date publications).

The five training modules parallel each chapter in the manual for workers. Each consists of a summary of the fundamental body of knowledge found in the manual, which sequentially enlarges the capacity of mental health counselors to participate in emergency and post-disaster assistance programs in unison with all other post-disaster governmental agencies. The instructor or trainer using this guide can choose the number and combination of training modules to be used according to the instruction to be offered, which in turn will be determined by their students' level of preparedness. The content of the guide can thus be adapted so that it is as narrow or as broad as needed in any given situation. In other words, by tailoring the modules, the guide can be expanded or reduced without loosing its focus.

Each module includes the following parts:

1. **Learning objectives:** Identifies the knowledge, skills, and attitudes that the student will acquire.
2. **Content summary:** The content of each module includes a summary of the more complete material presented in the worker's manual. The aim is to give trainers enough substance so that they can select the amounts necessary for their self-learning or for adaptation to the characteristics of their team members.
3. **Teaching resources:** Training aids to assist in presenting the content. Each module includes a number of pages can be made into transparencies or slides. The trainer will choose a few specific pages and make slides or transparencies appropriate for the students' previous level of knowledge (e.g., paraprofessionals). The teaching resources vary in level of sophistication, giving the teacher a number of choices. Videotapes on disasters can help illustrate content or be used in group exercises. Ideally, the videos should reflect the language, type of disaster, and culture of the region.
4. **Group work/exercises:** A number of examples are included that will assist the trainer in putting into practice the principles presented in the content. Before

each assignment, students and teacher should collaboratively identify the educational objectives and write them out. Again, they should reflect the characteristics of the population and the event.

5. **Reading list:** The articles have been selected to further enhance workers' knowledge, but they do not represent a complete bibliography on the subjects covered. Additional information on topics of special interest can be obtained through a computer search or from the Regional Disaster Information Center (CRID), Apartado Postal 3745-1000, San José, Costa Rica, telephone: 506-296-32-52, fax: 506-231-59-73, e-mail: crid@crid.or.cr, website: www.crid.or.cr.

Training manual and materials produced in the United States

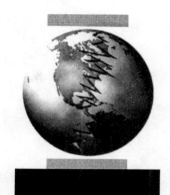

American Red Cross. *Disaster Mental Health Provider's Course.* Washington, D.C.: American Red Cross; April 1991. (ARC 3076A).

Faberow NL, Frederick CJ. *Training Manual for Human Service Workers in Major Disasters.* Rockville, Maryland: National Institute of Mental Health; 1978. (DHHS Publication No. (ADM) 86-538).

National Institute of Mental Health. *Field Manual for Human Service Workers in Major Disasters.* Rockville, Maryland: NIMH; 1978. (DHHS Publication No. (ADM) 87-537).

Hartsough DM, Myers DG. *Disaster Work and Mental Health: Prevention and Control of Stress Among Workers.* Rockville, Maryland: National Institute of Mental Health, 1985. (DHHS Publication No. (ADM) 87-1422).

Myers D. *Disaster Response and Recovery: A Handbook for Mental Health Professionals.* Washington, D.C.: U.S. Department of Health and Human Services, Center for Mental Health Services; 1994. (DHHS Publication No. (SMA) 94-3010).

Videos

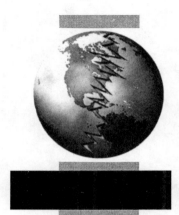

Beyond the Ashes. City of Berkeley Mental Health Division, California Department of Mental Health, National Institute of Mental Health, and Federal Emergency Management Agency; 1992.

Children and Trauma: The School's Response. California Department of Mental Health, National Institute of Mental Health, and Federal Emergency Management Agency; 1991. Available from Center for Mental Health Services, 5600 Fishers Lane, Room 16C-26, Rockville, MD 20857.

Disaster Psychology: Victim Response. University of Maryland Baltimore County, Catonsville, MD: Instructional Media Resources; 1985. 30-minute videotape.

Faces in the Fire: One Year Later. Santa Barbara County Department of Mental Health and Federal Emergency Management Agency; 1991. Available from Center for Mental Health Services, 5600 Fishers Lane, Room 16C-26, Rockville, MD 20857.

Human Response to Disaster: Training Emergency Service Workers. Rockville, Maryland: National Institute of Mental Health; 1984. Six 20-minute videotapes.

Hurricane Blues. South Carolina Department of Mental Health, National Institute of Mental Health, and Federal Emergency Management Agency. 1990. Available from Center for Mental Health Services, 5600 Fishers Lane, Room 16C-26, Rockville, MD 20857.

KEY CONCEPTS OF DISASTER MENTAL HEALTH*

1. No one who sees a disaster is untouched by it.
2. There are two types of disaster trauma.
3. Most people pull together and function during and after a disaster, but their effectiveness is diminished.
4. Disaster stress and grief reactions are a normal response to an abnormal situation.
5. Many emotional reactions of disaster survivors stem from *problems of living* brought about by the disaster.
6. Disaster relief procedures have been called "the second disaster."
7. Most people do not see themselves as needing mental health services following disaster and will not seek out such services.
8. Survivors may reject disaster assistance of all types.
9. Disaster mental health assistance is often more "practical" than "psychological" in nature.
10. Disaster mental health services must be uniquely tailored to the communities they serve.
11. Mental health staff need to set aside traditional methods, avoid the use of mental health labels, and use an active outreach approach to intervene successfully in disaster.
12. Survivors respond to active interest and concern.
13. Interventions must be appropriate to the phase of disaster.
14. Support systems are crucial to recovery.

* Source: Myers D. *Disaster Response and Recovery: A Handbook for Mental Health Professionals.* Washington, D.C.: U.S. Department of Health and Human Services, Center for Mental Health Services; 1994. (DHHS Publication No. (SMA) 94-3010).

Historical overview

Mental health role

Sociocultural characteristics

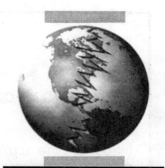

CHAPTER 1

■ TRAINING MODULE

Module 1:
Introduces the applied content of mental health participation in post-disaster programs.

■ WHY HAVE THIS MODULE?

To place in context the role of mental health workers within a multidisciplinary post-disaster setting

To present sociocultural guidelines for understanding post-disaster reactions in differing populations.

■ CONTENT

• Historical overview

• The mental health worker as a disaster assistance participant/ helper.

• Key sociocultural variables affecting post-disaster behavior.

◼◼ LEARNING OBJECTIVES

After participating in Module 1 the student will:

- Possess knowledge of key historical developments in the field of post-disaster intervention.
- Be able to identify the role, skills, and attitudes of the mental health worker within a multiagency and multidisciplinary post-disaster setting.
- Be able to identify the sociocultural factors influencing post-disaster reactions in the survivor population.
- Be able to identify the cultural diversity issues that may arise during assessment, crisis counseling, and post-disaster interventions.
- Recognize important similarities and differences between cultural groups.

◼◼ CONTENT SUMMARY

◼ HISTORICAL OVERVIEW

Important events in the development of disaster mental health programs in the United States are described as an example of how a country has responded to the needs of a population. If the training is taking place in another country, the trainer should obtain information on how that country has developed its post-disaster mental health systems and resources.

◼ MENTAL HEALTH ROLE

The role of the post disaster worker is evolving and restructuring its boundaries as more workers have an opportunity to acquire and share experiences in intervention worldwide. Most workers, who have no experience with disasters, must either acquire new techniques or shift their usual mode of work and theoretical focus to a new system of guidelines and at the same time develop the skills, knowledge, and attitudes needed to work with individuals who are not responding in a pathological way but are exhibiting normal reactions to an abnormal situation. A description of the appropriate skills and attitudes is provided.

◼ SOCIOCULTURAL CHARACTERISTICS

In a disaster, an awareness of different sociocultural populations will help workers assist survivors from diverse backgrounds. Therefore, content based on experience and knowledge of specific cultures from the region in which the disaster has occurred should be incorporated throughout the training process.

In different cultures behavior develops out of the many roles a survivor played before the disaster. This role was molded by status and economic position. It carries with it symbols of culturally defined expectations about the patterns of relationships and behavior within a particular social system. The array of roles and behaviors may be perceived differently by a worker from another culture. Differences in customs and languages, if ignored, lead to failure and frustration. In delivering services to persons of different racial and ethnic groups, language, and socioeconomic levels, it is essential that outreach efforts be channeled through representatives or facilities within their own cultural area.

A list of concepts is included to establish the basic principles of assisting a population from a different culture than that of the worker.

■■■ TEACHING RESOURCES

Suggestions for using the teaching resources in this training module:

a. The role of the mental health worker. A list of behavior categories identifying and contrasting the disaster mental health worker with a mental health clinician is presented and should be analyzed and discussed by the group as a review of content.

b. The "shift" process should be emphasized as a difficult process that requires continued awareness throughout all phases of the program.

c. A list of key variables describing the behavior of sub-populations should be identified within the populations affected by the disaster.

Bicultural communication problems should be identified so that workers become conscious of their own values, attitudes, and behavior toward survivors.

Note to Trainer: The following pages are ready to be used as transparencies, slides, or handouts.

THE ROLE OF THE MENTAL HEALTH WORKER AS A POST-DISASTER PARTICIPANT

Role definition

Functions

Skills

Responsibilities

Theoretical and practical guidelines to support their work with survivors

Attitudes

Decision-making and power

Professional boundaries vs. amorphous boundaries

Prioritization of needs and resources

Advocacy

Functions and role shift in the mental health profession

- Commonality with traditional knowledge
- Different and novel variety of functions
- New attitudes - co-professional
- Rhythm and timing - crisis contingencies
- Evolution in expectations and attitudes of non-mental health workers
- Disaster-assistance workers - responsibilities different from those of mental health workers
- Participatory and collaborative consultation

THE EFFECT OF SURVIVOR'S SOCIOECONOMIC LEVEL ON THE DEVELOPMENT OF PSYCHOLOGICAL SYMPTOMS AFTER A DISASTER

Many studies of the general population have shown that persons of low income and low educational levels are at higher risk for prolonged serious psychological problems than persons in higher socioeconomic classes.

- Persons at lower socioeconomic levels are more likely to seek medical than psychological treatment.

- Intensive outreach may be needed to reach these groups in times of emergency if they are to receive the care they need (NIMH 1983).

- People in middle- and upper-income levels are likely to be more aware of their problems and less resistant to accepting needed help.

- Upper-income persons may be less inclined than those in lower- and middle-income groups to welcome outreach and "free" services (NIMH 1983).

DEFINITION

Acculturation

The complex process of accommodation of the total cultural content: one dimensional and two dimensional. Capacity to keep one's own values while incorporating values of another culture comfortably.

**Behavior
perceived as
determined
by**

role-sociocultural
norms-sociocultural
self-concept-intrapsychic
interpersonal agreements-characteristic of bonds and loyalties

+

**Social
cognition**

intrapersonal-other people's cultural expectations
emotional attachments-personal priorities the value associated with perceived consequence of behavior

■ CULTURAL ISSUES

Trainers will have to identify the cultural groups within the survivor population and adapt their training approaches based on the knowledge they have or need to acquire to help the individuals affected by the disaster. Based on this knowledge, they will need to modify their skills to intervene and assist effectively in crisis counseling. The trainers will have to adapt the resources and exercises to cultural factors and practice approaches and attitudes with the assistance of teachers native to the area. The training should incorporate continuous supervision and awareness of the unique responses of different cultural groups.

■ OPERATIONAL GUIDELINES

Cultural variations in the manifestation and conceptualization of crisis responses need to be recognized and used to modify approaches to crisis counseling. As the services are organized, fully accessible outreach and culturally appropriate interventions should be offered. The concept of bridging—teaching and training multiethnic, multidisciplinary teams—should be planned for a community where survivors will represent diverse populations.

In teaching team members about a particular culture, the trainer should focus not only on beliefs and practices that may impinge on effective counseling, but also on adaptive strategies, strengths, and support elements in the community. Community outreach techniques have to be developed and become an integral aspect of the delivery of culturally appropriate services. As part of this outreach approach, characteristics of the social matrix, value and worldview, family structure, child-rearing practices, and sex role relationships should be taken into account.

Adding these areas of knowledge will facilitate or improve counselors' work with survivors in cultures different from their own and provide them with a transcultural perspective in the application of crisis counseling. This, in turn, will improve their interpretative skills by providing information that will enable the counselors to better understand the conceptual framework of the survivors and sharpen the interaction skills that will decrease survivors' culturally based resistance to accept assistance after the disaster.

The examination of belief systems, values, and cultural dimensions in a transcultural context will facilitate the development of a mode of perception that questions the "universality" of responses to trauma and will thus enable the counselor to seek alternate interpretations of behavior.

Any training model designed to foster cross-cultural effectiveness and sensitivity must recognize the compelling and central role of both religious belief and church affiliation in strengthening and promoting adaptive coping among survivors in the specific community where the disaster has struck. The importance of outreach and linkage with key religious figures should be emphasized, as many survivors may benefit from referral to religious institutions for advisory and support services.

The training model for effective and sensitive cross-cultural post-disaster counseling should incorporate the following content:

- Recognize the difference between race, culture, ethnicity, and related key concepts that will have an influence in responses to the effects of the disaster.
- Understand that, since most of our cultural learning takes place unconsciously, we grow up thinking that our values, beliefs, and behaviors are "right" and "natural."
- Understand that counselors should be aware of their own cultural learning as well as that of the survivors and recognize the differences.
- Become aware that cultural groups learn different patterns of thinking and perception.
- Become aware of how language influences thinking and behavior.
- Learn how certain values held by counselors of one culture may interfere with the counseling process when they are working with survivors of a different culture.
- Have increased cognitive awareness of and respect for the influence of culture on the survivor's beliefs, values, and behaviors.
- Understand that there is no one culture which has access to universal "truth." Beliefs, behaviors, and values are best viewed as being appropriate to the social and physical environment in which the culture has developed.

Benefits of this type of training:

Knowledge of Content

1. Significant increases in the counselor's cultural knowledge.
2. Significant decreases in the counselor's social, affective, and attitudinal distance from other cultures.
3. Significant increases in comprehension of and respect for cultural values.
4. Behavioral demonstration of significant increase in counseling effectiveness with survivors of different cultures.
5. Acquisition of a transcultural perspective to enable generalization of counseling skills across a variety of target populations used in an integrative manner that is relevant to survivors.

Knowledge of Skills

Traditionally, post-disaster workers have utilized counseling and service modalities which have been developed and applied almost exclusively with the values and frame of reference of the majority population. Professional practice has shown that many of these modalities lack certain critical applicability and success with minority and other populations. Modification of skill methods is an attempt to bridge the conceptual and operational gaps that exist between basic crisis counseling and counseling that is sensitive to the needs of minorities, for example, survivors who are foreigners or members of an indigenous group. To this end, the manual is designed to provide counselors with the opportunity to enhance their practical skills so that they can be simultaneously effective and supportive.

The following guidelines will help counselors introduce the modifications needed to adapt their basic counseling skills to diverse cultural survivors:

- Be aware of the ways in which multicultural differences between counselor and counselee affect the post-disaster crisis counseling process.
- Add post-disaster counseling skills to your repertoire which are most appropriate to the life experiences of the affected population.
- Recognize that all crisis workers are culturally conditioned to respond in certain ways in the counseling process (e.g., in terms of time orientation, relationship with survivors).
- Develop cross-cultural counseling skills and attitudes.
- Begin to make behavioral changes in your counseling style with multicultural survivors from ethnic groups other than your own.
- Increase your ability to choose appropriate questions, correctly interpret responses, and plan the most appropriate post-disaster treatment plan.
- Develop skill in handling beginnings and endings of cross-cultural post-disaster counseling sessions and relationships.
- Develop skill in handling direct requests for advice from survivors.
- Develop skill in handling requests for self-disclosure.
- Be able to handle expressions of distrust from a survivor of an ethnic background different from your own, and be able to differentiate this from paranoia.
- Develop skill in differentiating resistance from fear of transgressing a cultural norm.
- Develop skill in handling requests for referral to another mental health agency and assist in the linking process.
- Become aware of the problems which may arise in applying a crisis intervention technique developed for use within one specific culture to a survivor from a different culture.

■ GROUP WORK/EXERCISES

Exercise 1

The instructor asks the students to list differences between a mental health clinician and a post-disaster mental health worker.

Exercise 2

The instructor asks the students to list the problems they envision a mental health worker will have developing and carrying out the new role of emergency disaster worker.

Exercise 3

The instructor asks the students to discuss their own awareness of how different populations might respond to a disaster, including African-Americans, Hispanics/ Latinos, Asians, and Caribbean peoples.

■ HOW SPECIFIC CULTURAL AND RACIAL GROUPS AFFECT INTERVENTION DECISIONS — Discuss each point.

a. In recent years, disaster relief workers have emphasized the importance of socially and culturally appropriate interventions. Differences of custom and language, if ignored, lead to failure and frustration.
b. In delivering services to persons of different race or ethnicity, language, and socioeconomic levels, it is essential that outreach efforts be channeled through representatives or facilities within the subcultural area.

Migrant and refugee populations present special problems, especially when there is a large influx of a group into the disaster area. While the vast majority will surmount the stresses of departure from their cultures, many will require the skilled assistance of mental health workers.

Many members of minority groups do not seek help, partly because of culturally biased perceptions toward counseling and partly because of the inappropriateness and inaccessibility of services. Thus, when they do seek help, their problems are likely to be serious.

Where culturally sensitive post-disaster mental health services are available, survivors do use them. Successful services for these populations typically have the following characteristics: bilingual staff, integration of cultural patterns into counseling modes, involvement of the family and community in treatment, integration of the survivor into family and community systems, encouragement of the survivor's self-sufficiency, and cultural awareness training for counselors.

Exercise 4

Objective of this exercise:

1. To begin questioning the processes by which one infers the correlates and reasons for observable behavior (i.e., what does behavior represent, what does it mean?)
2. To analyze certain culture-normative behaviors against which individual behavior might be measured, understood, and supported.
3. To examine and understand one's own reaction to a time-limited crisis experience in a cultural setting different from that with which one ordinarily identifies.

Choose a case that highlights cultural differences and cast the post-disaster crisis counselor in an unfamiliar role-simulation of a survivor from another culture, so that the counselor becomes aware of his/her own culturally bound values in interpreting someone else's behavior.

EXERCISE 4

Please circle the number that you feel best described the counselor's behavior.

Performance Level

High - Low

1. Helps the survivor feel comfortable.   1   2   3
2. Defines purpose of the interview.   1   2   3
3. Clarifies own role as helping person.   1   2   3
4. Establishes rapport with survivors.   1   2   3
5. Uses appropriate vocabulary.   1   2   3
6. Responds appropriately to survivor's   1   2   3
   questions.
7. Ask facilitating questions.   1   2   3
8. Addresses the presenting problem   1   2   3
   appropriately.
9. Facilitates taking of important decisions.   1   2   3
10. Allows survivor expression with minimal   1   2   3
    inappropriate interruptions.
11. Has respectful and attentive manner.   1   2   3
12. Shows knowledge of resources to deal with   1   2   3
    with survivors' complaints and refers to
    appropriate agency.
13. Shows understanding of survivors' socio-   1   2   3
    cultural context in dealing with problems.
14. Conveys reassurance or hope that problems   1   2   3
    can be resolved.
15. Educates survivor in how to deal with   1   2   3
    problems related to the post-disaster
    reality.

Please answer the following as though you were a survivor.

16. How well did this counselor deal with your   1   2   3
    complaint?
17. How well did this counselor understand your   1   2   3
    problem?
18. How much would you want to return to this   1   2   3
    person if you needed other kinds of help?

EXERCISE 4:
CROSS-CULTURAL COMMUNICATION

Poor communication is often the result of multiple factors. Please indicate below the five items which you believe are the most serious barriers to effective cross-cultural communication.

1. Sender has poor knowledge of subject or is inadequately prepared.
2. Sender does not believe in message or approach behind it.
3. Receiver has poor knowledge of subject or is inadequately prepared.
4. Receiver is not interested in subject.
5. Sender or receiver is temporarily preoccupied.
6. Unintentional failure of people to say what they mean.
7. Sender and receiver have very different vocabularies, values, worldview.
8. Cultural differences between communicators set up social distance.
9. Socioeconomic differences between communicators.
10. Communicators have different assumptions.
11. Status differences (as leader-member) between communicators.
12. One of the communicators has negative or hostile reactions to the other.
13. One of the communicators tends to be a "yes man" to the other.
14. One or both parties is unintentionally miscommunicating.
15. Outside interference or distractions.
16. Pressure of time.
17. Inadequacy of words to express difficult concepts, relationships, or situations.
18. Same words have different meanings.
19. Inadequate feedback system.
20. Sender and receiver belong in different subgroups.
21. Differences in age between persons.
22. (Add any other you've identified.)

After you select five items that impede communication between a counselor and a survivor of different cultures, suggest methods to minimize the situation.

READING LIST

Ahearn, FL and Cohen, RE (eds.). *Disaster and mental health, an annotated bibliography.* Washington, D.C.: U.S. Government Printing Office; 1985.

Austin L. In the wake of Hugo: the role of the psychiatrist. *Psychiatric Annals* 1991; 21(9):502-527.

Baum A, Solomon SD, Ursano R J. Emergency /disaster studies: practical conceptual, and methodological issues. In: Wilson JP and Raphael B (eds.). *The international handbook of traumatic stress syndromes.* New York: Plenum Press Inc.; 1992.

Cohen R (1972). Principles of preventive mental health programs for ethnic minority populations. The acculturation of Puerto Ricans to the United States. *American Journal of Psychiatry* 1972;128(12).

Cohen R, Culp C, Genser S. *Human problems in major disasters: a training curriculum for emergency medical personnel.* Washington, D.C.: US Government Printing Office; 1987. (DHHS publication no (ADM) 88-1505).

Cohen RE Training mental health professionals to work with families in diverse cultural contexts. In Austin L (ed.). *Responding to disaster: a guide for mental health professionals.* Washington, D.C.: APPI; 1992: 69-80.

Cohen RE Stressors: Migration and acculturation to American society. In: Gaviria M, Arana J (eds.). *Health and behavior: research agenda for Hispanics.* Chicago: University of Illinois; 1987. (Simón Bolívar Research Monograph Series No. 1).

Cole M, Bruner J. Cultural differences and inferences about psychological process. *American Psychologist* 1971; 26: 867-876.

Dana, RH. *Multicultural assessment perspectives for professional psychology.* Boston: Allyn and Bacon; 1993.

Davidson JRT, Foa EB (eds.). *Posttraumatic stress disorder: DSM-IV and beyond.* Washington, D.C.: American Psychiatric Press; 1993.

Disaster Relief Act, Public Law 93-288 (93rd Congress); 1974.

Figley C (ed.) *Trauma and its wake.* New York: Brunner/Mazel; 1985.

Folkman S, Lazarus RS, Pimley S, Novack J. Age differences in stress and coping processes. *Psychology and Aging* 1987; 2: 171-184.

Gelford D. Ethnicity, aging and mental health. *International Journal of Aging and Human Development* 1979-1980; 10(31): 289-298.

Green BL. Traumatic stress and disaster: mental health effects and factors influencing adaptation. In: Lie Mac E , Nadelson C (eds) and Davidson JRT, McFarlane A(section editors). *International Review of Psychiatry* (Vol II). Washington, D.C.: APA Press, Inc. and American Psychiatric Association; 1993.

Green BL . Defining trauma: terminology and generic stressor dimensions. *Journal of Applied Social Psychology* 1990; 20:1632-1642.

Henderson G (ed.). *Understanding and counseling ethnic minorities.* Springfield, Illinois: Charles C. Thomas Publisher, Ltd.; 1980.

Hodkinson PE, Stewart M. *Coping with catastrophe: a handbook of disaster management.* New York: Routledge; 1991.

Horowitz MJ. *Stress response syndrome* (2nd ed.) Northvale, New Jersey: Jason Aronson, Inc.; 1986.

Jackson G. The emergence of a Black perspective in counseling. *The Journal of Negro Education* 1977;46(3): 230-253.

Jones D J. Secondary disaster victims: the emotional effects of recovery and identifying human remains. *American Journal of Psychiatry* 1985; 142(3):303-307.

Kitano HHL, Matsushima N. Counseling Asian Americans. In: Pedersen P, Draguns J, Lonner W, Trimble J (eds.). *Counseling across cultures* (Second Edition). Honolulu: The University of Hawaii Press; 1981.

Mitchell H. Counseling Black students: a model in response to the need for relevant counselor training programs. In: Atkinson DR, Morten G, Sue DW (eds.). *Counseling American minorities.* Dubuque, Iowa: Wm. C. Brown Company Publishers; 1979.

Pedersen P. Culturally inclusive and culturally exclusive models of counseling. In: Pedersen P, Draguns J, Lonner W, Trimble J (eds.). *Counseling across cultures* (Second Edition). Honolulu: The University of Hawaii Press; 1981.

Raphael B. *When disaster strikes: how individuals and communities cope with catastrophe.* New York: Basic Books; 1986.

Ruiz RA, Padilla AM. Counseling Latinos. In: Atkinson DR, Morten G, Sue DW (eds.). *Counseling American minorities.* Dubuque, Iowa: Wm. C. Brown Company Publishers; 1979.

Scott M J. Counseling for trauma and posttraumatic stress disorder. In: Palmer S, McMahon G (eds.). *Handbook of counseling.* London: Routledge; 1997.

Scott M J, Stradling SG. *Counseling for post-traumatic stress disorder.* London: Sage Publications; 1992.

Sue DW, Sue S. Counseling Chinese-Americans. In: Atkinson DR, Morten G, Sue DW (eds.). *Counseling American minorities.* Dubuque, Iowa: Wm. C. Brown Company Publishers; 1979.

Toupin E. Counseling Asians: Psychotherapy in the context of racism and Asian American history. *American Journal of Orthopsychiatry* 1980; 50(1): 76-80.

Trimble JE. Value differentials and their importance in counseling American Indians. In: Pedersen P, Draguns J, Lonner W, Trimble J (eds.). *Counseling across cultures* (Second Edition). Honolulu: The University of Hawaii Press; 1981.

van der Kolk B (ed). *Psychological Trauma.* Washington, D.C.: American Psychiatric Press; 1987.

Wilson JP, Raphael B (eds.). *International handbook of traumatic stress syndromes.* New York: Plenum Press; 1993.

Wolf ME, Mosnaim AD (eds.). *Post-traumatic stress disorder: etiology, phenomenology, and treatment.* Washington, D.C.: American Psychiatric Press; 1990.

A review of basic and applied knowledge for the development of post-disaster intervention guidelines

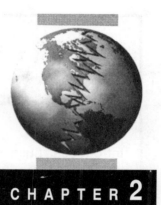

CHAPTER 2

■ TRAINING MODULE

Module 2:
Introduces "building-block knowledge" to guide post-disaster intervention.

■ WHY HAVE THIS MODULE?

To present the basic content for understanding survivor reactions and formulating post-disaster interventions.

■ CONTENT

Basic concepts of mental health:

- Stressor/stress reactions

- Coping and adaptation

- Loss and mourning

- Social support

- Crisis response and resolution

■■■ LEARNING OBJECTIVES

At the end of the presentation students will:

- Be able to identify theories of stressor/stress response, loss and mourning, social support systems, crisis response and resolution.
- Be able to identify the basic building blocks of knowledge to guide post-disaster intervention.
- Possess the knowledge needed to recognize survivors' reactions and formulate post-disaster interventions.

■■■ CONTENT SUMMARY

This module presents additional basic knowledge that supports the understanding of survivors' post-disaster behavior as an expression of their response to trauma. The group of responses that have been selected to aid in the understanding of post-disaster behavior has been found to be present in survivors as a universal reaction worldwide. Nevertheless, it is important to emphasize that, although basic human reactions to trauma are universal, facial and bodily reactions, emotionality, expressiveness, and voice tone are influenced by cultural factors. The discrete areas of knowledge will help reinforce the knowledge which experienced workers already possess but which will be used differently in post-disaster intervention. Inexperienced workers will acquire the knowledge they need to assist survivors. All the areas of knowledge relate to the reactions of survivors coping with a changed environment.

The information presented in the following areas reviews known content but focuses it toward identifying, recognizing, and understanding human responses after a disaster:

- Stressor/stress reactions
- Coping and adaptation
- Loss, grieving, and mourning
- Social support systems
- Crisis response and resolution

■■■ TEACHING RESOURCES

Suggestions for using the teaching resources in Chapter 2:

a. Social Readjustment Rating Scale: This document can be used to identify a list of stressful events that may occur after a disaster. It will illustrate the painful process faced by survivors.

b. Several documents define in more detail the conceptual systems approach to understand human adaptation mechanisms.

c. The stress model developed by the Institute of Medicine illustrates the interaction of variables that enter into play after a disaster. The principal contribution of this model is its emphasis on identifying reactions versus consequences (long-lasting with possible pathological outcomes).

Note to Trainer: The following pages are ready to be used as transparencies, slides, or handouts.

SOCIAL READJUSTMENT RATING SCALE

Rank	Life Event	Mean Value	Rank	Life Event	Mean Value
1.	Death of Spouse	100	21.	Foreclosure of Mortgage or Loan	30
2.	Divorce	73	22.	Change in Responsibilities at Work	29
3.	Marital Separation	65	23.	Son or Daughter Leaving Home	29
4.	Prison Sentence or Jail Term	63	24.	Trouble with In-Laws	29
5.	Death of a Close Family Member	63	25.	Outstanding Personal Achievement	28
6.	Personal Illness or Injury	53	26.	Wife Begin or Stop Work	26
7.	Marriage	50	27.	Begin or End School	26
8.	Fired at Work	47	28.	Change in Living Conditions	25
9.	Marital Reconciliation	45	29.	Revision of Personal Habit	24
10.	Retirement	45	30.	Trouble with Boss	23
11.	Change in Health of Family Member	44	31.	Change in Work House or Conditions	20
12.	Pregnancy	40	32.	Change in Residence	20
13.	Sex Difficulties	39	33.	Change in Schools	20
14.	Gain of New Family Member	39	34.	Change in Recreation	19
15.	Business Readjustment	39	35.	Change in Church Activities	19
16.	Change in Financial State	38	36.	Change in Social Activities	18
17.	Death of a Close Friend	37	37.	Mortgage or Loan Less Than $10,000	17
18.	Change to Different Line of Work	36	38.	Change in Sleeping Habits	16
19.	Change in Number of Arguments with Spouse	35	39.	Change in Number of Family Get-togethers	15
20.	Mortgage Over $10,000	31	40.	Change in Eating Habits	15
			41.	Vacation	13
			42.	Christmas	12
			43.	Minor Violations of the Law	11

From Holmes and Rahe. Social readjustment rating scale. In: Dohrenwend BS, Dohrenwend BP (eds.). *Stressful life events: their nature and effects.* New York: Wiley Interscience; 1974: Table 3, p. 216.

REACTIONS TO AN UNPREDICTABLE ENVIRONMENT

An individual placed within an environment where his/her "usual" behavior no longer leads to a formerly predictable outcome nor has an impact (control) on that environment will experience an increased level of anxiety—acute, constant, or chronic. This human reaction affects the internal functions which controls behavior (physiologic and psychologic) which in turn increases susceptibility to:

• ACTING OUT

• DISTORTED BEHAVIOR

• ILLNESS

• PSYCHIC DISORGANIZATION

BIO-PSYCHO-SOCIO-CULTURAL MODEL

OFFERS A CONCEPTUAL BASIS FOR UNDERSTANDING POST-DISASTER REACTIONS AND COUNSELING INTERVENTION

The bio-psycho-socio-cultural model is a scientific model constructed to take into account all the dimensions of an organism (plus its functions) within an environment. It is based on a systems approach incorporating human relations expressed in psychological and behavioral terms.

THE BIO-PSYCHO-SOCIO-CULTURAL SYSTEM

1. The organism is a dynamic, evolving system of information exchange and processing. It changes and shifts after receiving the early signals of the disaster.

2. It exists in an ever-changing environment where information transfer occurs within and between the brain and the environment. The impact on the senses (visual, auditory) sets up different processes that influence perception.

3. The interrelationship of subsystems consists of a large variety of communication signals transmitted in a regular or irregular rhythmic manner. Most of the signals are unfamiliar and increase irregular rythms.

4. The organism is an intricate communication system of information exchanged by means of signals coming from external and internal sources and affecting the rhythm of these communication signals (neurological, hormonal, endocrine). These biological systems shift affecting behavior after the disaster.

5. Stressful experience perturbs these rhythms and affects function, at times disorganizing them. This helps us understand some changes of behavior post-disaster.

6. Function is a unifying and dynamic concept that focuses on an integrated approach of the organism in its world. The patterns of physiology and behavior are inextricable. Coordinated, so that any disorganization affects function.

7. Any perturbation of one component of the organism will lead to a change in function, which forms the basis of stress response theory. Supports our understanding of disaster response.

8. Specific integrated, coordinated, and appropriate responses to each stressful experience occur. At times, depending on individual characteristics, these responses may be inappropriate, excessive, or inadequate, in which case symptoms may occur during certain phases post-disaster.

* Key concepts supporting an understanding of survivors as documented in Weiner H. *Perturbing the Organism: The Biology of Stressful Experience* Chicago: University of Chicago Press; 1992.

CONCEPTUAL FRAMEWORK
FOR "STRESS RESPONSE"

Interaction Between:

Stressor (X) = Reactions (Y) + Consequence (Z)

Sequelae to Reactions Depend on Characteristic of Stressor, Person Resources, and Task Required

Nature of Social Environment

$$\downarrow$$

(Outcome)

(Growth, Temporary Difficulty, Trauma)

Function of

$$\downarrow$$

1. Pervasiveness/persistence of stressor;
2. Life timing;
3. Reactive resources;
4. Opportunity/ability to act on environment;
5. Meaning attached to the experience

Institute of Medicine. *Research on Stress and Human Health.* Washington, D.C.: National Academy Press; 1981. [Report of a study by the Institute of Medicine, Division of Mental Health and Behavior].

CONCEPTUAL FRAMEWORK
FOR "STRESS RESPONSE"
(Continued)

DEFINITIONS:

• Stressors (Activators) - Events or conditions that elicit physical or psychosocial reactions (in a particular individual under specific conditions) - intensity, quantity, temporal pattern relationships.

• Reactions - Biological or psychosocial responses of an individual to a stressor - vary in intensity, effectiveness, or appropriateness of response within temporal patterns - temporary, transitory, difficulties.

• Consequences - Physical or psychosocial results of prolonged/cumulative effect of the reaction (some are positive/favorable).

• Mediators - Filters and modifiers that define the context in which the stressor-reaction-consequence (X-Y-Z) sequence occurs - Produces individual variations in the X-Y-Z sequence. They can be biologic, psychologic, social. Social support systems facilitate the development of coping strategies that help people contain distress within tolerable limits, maintain self-esteem, preserve interpersonal relationships, meet the requirement of new situations.

STRESSOR-STRESS RESPONSE

- Stressors are intense stimuli that arouse the central nervous system, prompting it to "kick in" a specific psychophysiologic response of the organism programmed for survival.

- Initial response of "fight-flight preservation" {systems} impacts on other biologic systems of organism.

- These processes, in turn, energize unique individual behaviors that vary depending on (1) personality, (2) competence, (3) past experience (historical), and (4) cognitive interpretation of the event

- Length and strength of the impact will influence psychophysiologic reactions expressed as behavior, feeling, ideas, and somatic signs.

CONCEPT OF "PSYCHOSOCIAL STRESSOR"

Interpersonal relationships affect intrapsychic-biological states through a psychosocial process.

Stressor stimulates emotional arousal which is associated with biologic reaction of stress, stimulating adaptive-coping reactions that lead to effective dealing with the environment and human relationships and helping us meet our expectations.

BASIC CONCEPTUAL FRAMEWORK
BIO-PSYCHO-SOCIAL
ORGANISM

Support systems (mediators-regulators)

Assistance (at every level) to the individual in the aftermath of a disaster, person-to-person exchange.

- Provide support for identification

- Exchange of helpful information

- Opportunity to share coping techniques

- Support increased sense of worth

- Reinforcement for change and maintenance of effort (feedback on performance)

- Provide concrete aid and serve as advocates

- Problem-solving options and prioritization of solutions

- Support activity, support empowerment in the face of adverse conditions

COPING
(CONTENDING)

Coping is the behavior that protects us from becoming psychologically and physiologically disorganized.

Coping usually incorporates action-oriented behavior responses. It also employs cognitive, emotional, and perceptual appraisal processes.

1. May attempt to change the source of the stress.

2. May attempt to redefine the threat situation (meaning, degree of severity).

3. Attempts to find accommodation and compromise (passive acceptance; resignation; religious beliefs; destiny).

REPERTOIRE OF EFFECTIVE COPING SKILLS

1. Ability to orient oneself rapidly

2. Planning of decisive action

3. Mobilization of emergency problem-solving mechanisms

4. Appropriate use of assistance resources

5. Ability to deal simultaneously with the affective dimensions of the experience and the tasks that must be carried out

6. Appropriate expression of painful emotions

7. Acknowledgement of pain, without obsessing over troubled feelings

8. Development of strategies (contingency plans) to convert uncertainty into manageable risk—"process of situational mastery" (worry work/rehearsal for life change stress)

9. Acknowledgement of increased dependency needs and seeking, receiving, and using assistance

10. Tolerance of uncertainty without resorting to impulsive action

11. Reaction to environmental challenges (repertoire of "active mastery skills") and recognition of their positive value for growth

12. Use of non-destructive defenses and modes of tension relief to cope with anxiety

NEGATIVE COPING

1. Excessive denial, withdrawal, retreat, avoidance, frequent use of fantasy, poor reality testing

2. Impulsive behavior, venting rage on weaker individuals and creating scapegoats

3. Over-dependent, clinging, counter-dependent behavior, inability to evoke "caring" feelings from others

4. Emotional suppression, possibly leading to "hopeless-helpless-giving up" syndrome

5. Use of hyperritualistic behavior with no purpose

6. Fatigue and poor regulation of rest-work cycle

7. Addiction

8. Inability to use support systems

CRISIS THEORY - DEFINITION

"State of Crisis" - The organism is in a temporary, state of disequilibrium. precipitated by a stressor characterized as "inescapable". An intense situation that overwhelms our usual coping mechanisms.

- There is disruption of the usual "steady state" patterns— biologic, psychologic, cognitive, behavioral, interpersonal, social (emotional fluctuation).

- The situation can be an overwhelming concrete disaster or a subtle symbolic event linked to emotionally laden meaning that amplifies and distorts responses to reality events. We may also go into crisis over an anticipated event.

- Past, present, and future may blur, predisposing to, precipitating, and perpetuating a crisis.

- The stressor precipitates an intense situation that overwhelms the individual's usual coping mechanisms.

- A disruption of the usual "steady state" patterns— biologic, psychologic, cognitive, behavioral, interpersonal, and social patterns keep fluctuating over time toward a final equilibrium (individual variations).

■■■ GROUP WORK/EXERCISES

Group activity

Exercise 1. Show a film that presents disaster workers in action.

The film should show actual scenes from various disasters, including a flood, torna-do, and hurricane, with disaster workers functioning in various settings. Before showing it, ask the students to do the following:

- Let yourself identify with the experience of individuals in the film. See whom you identify with most strongly.
- Pay particular attention to the disaster workers in the film. What do you think it would be like to be in the various roles portrayed in the film?

Following the film, these questions might be used for discussion:

- Which scenes in the film affected you most? What were your feelings as you watched those scenes?
- Whom did you identify with in the film? What do you imagine it would have been like for you to be in their place?
- Which disaster workers did you identify with in the film? What do you think it would have been like to be in their roles?

Exercise 2. Material required: newsprint and felt-tipped pens, or blackboard and chalk.

Ask workers to list characteristic reactions and how to identify them:

a) Stress-response
b) Crisis reactions
c) Bereavement - initial phase - last phase
d) Coping - healthy and unhealthy

Exercise 3. Have workers tell their own experiences of how support systems assisted them in coping with a crisis.

Exercise 4. Stress response reactions

Present the following vignette to the students.

The situation of Mr. M., a 38-year-old salesman who had suffered severe injuries and lost his wife and only child in a major flood in the Midwestern United States, exemplifies a stress reaction to loss of loved ones, home, and job. Mr. M. was interviewed on the second day after the disaster. He had objected to some routine questioning about what he had lost, aimed at finishing his loss record documentation. When faced with the concrete task of describing the recent events, he broke down and started to cry. He composed himself in a few minutes, excused himself, and tried to explain how "strange" it was for him to feel tense and frightened all the time. He related this condition directly to the time he became aware of the flooding waters and to the consequences that followed. He described difficulty in swallowing and feelings of dread whenever anyone approached him. He could not concentrate enough to understand what people asked him. Instead, he became aware of his heart "racing" and his stomach contracting, and he experienced heightened feelings of irritability. He felt he could not stand another demand or intrusion into his life and wanted to be left alone. Everything was too much of an effort for him. He believed the "doctors" were efficient but cold and insensitive and that they added to his stress.

Questions:

1) Identify the physiologic and psychological reactions.
2) What stage of response can be identified by these signs?

Exercise 5: Life events

An example of a precipitous change in a life situation is highlighted by the following story, told during a recovery effort after a hurricane. A 48-year-old mother of two adolescents, recently divorced, was trapped in her car by fallen electrical wires and had suffered severe burns. She had to remain in that dangerous situation for over seven hours until the rescue team extricated her. She was brought to the hospital where she found out that her neighborhood had been severely damaged. No one, however, could inform her whether her two children were safe or tell her to which shelter they had been taken. For several hours she tried to find out, but due to road conditions, disrupted phone lines, and the other priorities of the few disaster workers, she was unable to get information. When interviewed, she expressed anxiety and shock at how she was being "pushed around." Her speech was rambling; she repeated over and over how she should never have left her children alone. She already felt that the divorce had been traumatic enough to them and now, again, she felt that she was a bad mother. Her sense of helplessness, anguish, disorientation, self-accusation, and continuous and frantic attempts to find out where her children were, coupled with her refusal to listen to or accept any explanations, reflect the first cycle of crisis behavior.

Questions:

1) Identify the physiologic and psychological reactions.
2) What stage of response can be identified by these signs? ■

READING LIST

Cohen S, McKay G. Social support, stress and the buffering hypothesis: a theoretical analysis. In: Baum A, Singer JE, Taylor SE (eds.). *Handbook of psychology and health*, Vol. 4 Hillsdale, New Jersey: Lawrence Erlbaum; 1984: pp. 253-267.

Cook JD, Bickman L. Social support and psychological symptomatology following natural disaster. *Journal of Traumatic Stress* 1990;3:541-556.

Hobfoll SE, Freedy JR. The availability and effective use of social support. *Journal of Social and Clinical Psychology* 1990; 9:91-103.

Horowitz MJ. *Stress response syndromes*. 2nd edition. Northvale, New Jersey: Jason Aronson; 1986.

Lazarus RS, Folkman S. *Stress, appraisal, and coping.* New York: Springer; 1984.

Lindemann E. Symptomatology and management of acute grief. *American Journal of Psychiatry* 1944;101:141-148.

Solomon SE. Enhancing social support for disaster victims. In: Sowder B (ed.). *Disasters and mental health: selected contemporary perspectives.* Washington, D.C.: Government Printing Office; 1985: pp. 107-121. (DHHS Publication No. (ADM) 85-1421).

Warheit GJ A propositional paradigm for estimating the impact of disaster in mental health. In: Sowder B (ed.). *Disasters and mental health: selected contemporary perspectives.* Washington, D.C.: Government Printing Office; 1985: pp. 196-214. (DHHS Publication No. (ADM) 85-1421).

Weiner H. *Perturbing the organism: the biology of stressful experience.* Chicago: University of Chicago Press; 1992.

Wilkinson CB. Aftermath of a disaster: the collapse of the Hyatt Regency Hotel skywalks. *American Journal of Psychiatry* 1983; 140(9): 1134-1139.

Developmental stages of survivor behavior

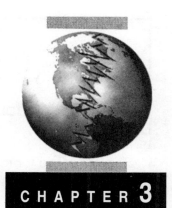

CHAPTER **3**

■ TRAINING MODULE

Module 3:

Sets the stage for recognizing the crisis response and adaptive behavior of survivors across post-disaster time phases.

■ WHY HAVE THIS MODULE?

To systematically categorize behavior processes through time phases.

■ CONTENT

Presents a composite grid to show the developmental stages of survivor behavior.

▌▌▌ LEARNING OBJECTIVES

After participating in Module 3 the students will:

- Be aware of behavior, thinking, and feelings of survivors with the passage of time post-disaster.
- Be able to conceptualize the sequences of changes as the survivor adapts to different stages of the disaster.

▌▌▌ CONTENT SUMMARY

This module presents a description of survivors' responses as they process their emotions through the different post-disaster time phases. The developmental sequence is similar to that which occurs in clinical resolution of crisis, trauma, and bereavement. Although the reaction sequences are not of fixed duration and flexible approaches are necessary, there appears to be a guiding developmental sequence to crisis resolution. The confounding influences that alter the sequence of responses are labeled the "secondary disaster," which consists of all the bureaucratic and reconstructive procedures that survivors must contend with after the disaster, coupled with their personal problems: loss of employment, marital problems, physical illness, etc.

Each phase of the process will necessitate different teaching content to enable mental health workers to help survivors deal with whatever stage of emotional response they are in when they are first seen by a worker. Each post-disaster phase will require different approaches by the worker.

Each phase—threat, impact, recoil, early aftermath, and late aftermath—is described from four perspectives: biological, psychological, interpersonal, and sociocultural. Examples of behavioral defenses are also given.

▌▌▌ TEACHING RESOURCES

Suggestions for the use the teaching resources in this module:

a) The time dimension of disaster: Dividing and labeling timeframes in the sequence of a disaster has become common practice in the field of disaster mental health. Each frame has specific characteristics that aid in defining the responses and planning for assistance. Different authors have labeled these frames with different names.

b) The sequences of observed and documented responses and defense mechanisms are presented in three pages to offer the student a rapid overview of the processes through which survivors pass as they adapt to their new environment. Where no data are available, the spaces have been left empty, but can be filled in as more information becomes available.

Note to Trainer: The following pages are ready to be used as transparencies, on slides, or handouts.

THE TIME DIMENSION OF DISASTER

Stages of Disaster

Pre-Disaster Conditions	1	2	3	4	5	6	7
	Warning	Threat	Impact	Inventory	Rescue	Remedy	Recovery

SOURCE: Reprinted from Powell JW. An introduction to the natural history of disaster. In: Wettenhall RL. *Bushfire Disaster: An Australian Community in Crisis.* Sydney: Angus and Robertson; 1975.

ANTICIPATION OF DISASTER: WARNINGS AND RESPONSE

1. Declining urgency, vigilance, and preparedness, but continued belief in reality of disaster impact.

2. Declining urgency and vigilance, belief that prediction was probably a false alarm.

3. Accumulating anxiety and fear, with defensive denial of danger.

4. Accumulating personal tension translated into anger and resentment, felt especially toward authorities.

5. Familiarization with and sensitization to signs of danger and appreciation of its implications.

6. Greater preparation for the eventual emergency, as a result of rehearsals and drills in response to early and repeated warnings.

DEVELOPMENTAL PHASES OF BEHAVIOR IN NATURAL DISASTERS				
	THREAT		**IMPACT**	
	Behavior	**Defense Mechanism**	**Behavior**	**Defense Mechanism**
Biological			Changes in neurochemical levels in the body Fatigue Exhaustion Over-activity	Health Nutrition Effect on immune response
Psychological	Superstition Rumor Confusion Passive-Negative High sense of invulnerability Humor	Denial Displacement Reaction formation	Centrality Reversal of usual behavior Fear Anxiety Cognitive clouding	Denial Action-focus Passivity Docility
Interpersonal	Helping Planning Shopping Community activity "Worry Work"		Helplessness Self-isolation Docility Dependency Indecisiveness Scapegoating Guilt	Extending support Grouping Independent position Rigid behavior
Sociocultural	Fatalism Religious activities Community preparedness	Human systems 1. Effective 2. Non-effective Fragmented	Family Ties Strengthening of religious feelings Influence of myths	Status Role strength Social support Primary relationships

DEVELOPMENTAL PHASES OF BEHAVIOR IN NATURAL DISASTERS (continued)				
	RECOIL		EARLY AFTERMATH	
	Behavior	Defense Mechanism	Behavior	Defense Mechanism
Biological	Insomnia Psychosomatic problems Irritability		Health aftermath, illness, injuries	
Psychological	Hyperactivity Underactivity Grief-Mourning Depression Narcissistic sensitivity Anxiety	Problem-solving Flexibility Denial Fantasy Repression Action-oriented	Return to normal function Less than normal function Resignation (pathological resolution) (Fixated in ambivalent emotion)	
Interpersonal	Easily "hurt" Difficulty in sharing Competition Frustration w/bureaucracy	Extending support Altruism Hoarding Rationalization Reaction-formation	Relations with job/family Reach different levels of accommodation	Use of usual defenses
Sociocultural	Traditional -stronger -weaker Religious activities			Increased/decreased use of legal & religious systems Greater use of medical systems

LATE AFTERMATH

A percentage of the population will continue to show:

PHYSIOLOGICAL

- Recurrent memory of events/hypersensitivity to sounds
- Flashbacks of traumatic moments
- Sleep disturbances/nightmares
- Tiredness/apathy/lack of motivation
- Anger/frustration/irritability
- Increase of psychosomatic problems
- Increased use of drugs/alcohol

PSYCHOLOGICAL

- Suicidal ideas
- Sense of helplessness/lack of control
- Lack of faith in future solutions
- Crying spells
- Depression
- Lack of tolerance/resentment
- Anticipatory fear of new disaster

SOCIAL

- Continuing problems with individuals from the private/ government/reconstruction sectors
- Problems with landlords
- Living in overcrowded homes/trailers
- Increase in domestic violence and gangs
- Traffic problems
- Lack of programs for children
- Increase in family tension

■■■ GROUP WORK/EXERCISES

Have trainees watch a film or video and identify the emotional reactions of survivors during the threat and impact phases. Assign each individual an observation role (survivor, worker). Ask them to share their observations with the group.

The following series of videos can be used for this module. All can be obtained from the U.S. Department of Health and Human Services, Center for Mental Health Services.

Human Response to Disaster: Training Emergency Service Workers
Diane Garaventa Myers, William T. O'Callahan, and Jack Peuler. Produced by the National Institute of Mental Health and state of California Department of Mental Health, in cooperation with the Federal Emergency Management Agency. Six 20-minute video-cassettes:

1. *Understanding Disaster and Disaster-Related Behavior*
2. *Impact and Rescue Phases: Issues and Interventions*
3. *Early Recovery Phases: Issues and Interventions*
4. *Late-Phase Recovery (2 months to 1 year): Issues and Interventions*
5. *Children and Disaster*
6. *Disaster Response Personnel: Stress and Coping Techniques* start new paragraph
This last video will provide trainers with an overview of stress and coping techniques for emergency workers. It discusses stressors affecting disaster workers, types of accidents that are especially critical or traumatic, phases of worker reactions to emergencies, stress symptoms of workers during and after impact, and helpful mental health interventions. It emphasizes and details the technique of debriefing.

Suggestions for Use

This series of videotapes can be used as a whole or in segments to provide introductory lecture material for both mental health and emergency workers.

Exercise 1: Post-disaster response in the first few hours

Present this example to the group, adjusting it as necessary to the cultural setting of the disaster.

An example of a precipitous change in a life situation is highlighted by the following story, told during a recovery effort after a hurricane. A 48-year-old mother of two adolescents, recently divorced, was trapped in her car by fallen electrical wires and had suffered severe burns. She had to remain in that dangerous situation for over seven hours until the rescue team extricated her. She was brought to the hospital where she found out that her neighborhood had been severely damaged. No one, however, could inform her whether her two children were safe or tell her to which shelter they had been taken. For several hours she tried to find out, but due to road conditions, disrupted phone lines, and the other priorities of the few disaster workers, she was unable to get information. When interviewed, she expressed anxiety and shock at how she was being "pushed around." Her speech was rambling; she repeated over and over how she should never have left her children alone. She already felt that the divorce had been traumatic enough to them and now, again, she felt that she was a bad mother. Her sense of helplessness, anguish, disorientation, self-accusation, and continuous and frantic attempts to find out where her children were, coupled with her refusal to listen to or accept any explanations, reflect the first cycle of crisis behavior.

Discussion: Ask the group to identify the psychological and physiological reactions of this survivor.

Divide the group into small subgroups. Ask each group to write a 5-minute script of a family situation describing what they might find following a disaster:

a) first week in a shelter
b) first month in a tent
c) third month in temporary housing
d) ninth month in permanent housing

The script should involve a worker and a group or family of survivors. A dialogue and description of the setting should be included.

Ask the participants to act out their scripts. A constructive analysis and discussion should follow. (This same situation will be used as a group exercise in Module 4 to practice intervention modalities).

Exercise 2: Family post-disaster response

Present the video *Hurricane Blues* * or another video illustrating the post-disaster interaction between a father, a mother, and teenaged children.

---

* South Carolina Department of Mental Health, National Institute of Mental Health, and Federal Emergency Management Agency. 1990. Available from Center for Mental Health Services, 5600 Fishers Lane, Room 16C-26, Rockville, MD 20857.

I. Divide the group into subgroups and ask each to list the following based on their observations of the disaster survivors in the video:

a) Emotional expressions
b) Behavior of family members
c) Dynamic interaction
   1. Between the children
   2. Between the adults
   3. Between children and adults

II. As a group, list the objectives of intervention to assist the family.

III. Pick one objective and role-play the intervention technique.

Stop the tape before the counselor presentation and proceed with the exercise. After the exercise is completed, play the counselor presentation and discuss. ■

READING LIST

Carlson EB. *Trauma assessments.* New York: Guilford Publications; 1997.

Cohen RE. Developmental phases of children's reactions following natural disaster. *Journal of the World Association of Emergency and Disaster Medicine* 1986(1-4):89-95.

Cohen RE. Reacciones individuales ante desastres naturales. *Boletín de la Organizacion Panamericana de la Salud.* April 1985:171-180.

Gavalya AS. Reactions to the Mexican earthquake: case vignettes. *Hospital Community Psychiatry* 1987;38:1327-1330.

Green BL. Traumatic stress and disaster: mental health effects and factors influencing adaptation. In: Lie Mac E , Nadelson C (eds) and Davidson JRT, McFarlane A *(*section editors). *International Review of Psychiatry* (Vol II). Washington, D.C.: APA Press, Inc. and American Psychiatric Association; 1993.

Laube J, Murphy S. *Perspectives on disaster recovery.* Norwalk, Connecticut: Appleton- Century-Crofts; 1985.

Madakasira S, O'Brien KF. Acute post-traumatic stress disorder in victims of a natural disaster. *Journal of Nervous and Mental Disorders* 1987;175:286-290.

Murphy SA. An explanatory model of recovery from disaster loss. *Research in Nursing and Health* 1989;12:67-76.

Myers D. Disaster response and recovery: a handbook for mental health professionals. Rockville, Maryland: Center for Mental Health Services: 1994.

Rapael, B. Mental health responses in a decade of disasters: Australia 1974-1983. *Hospital and Community Psychiatry* 1987;38(12):1331-1337.

Rundell RJ, Ursano JR. Psychiatric responses to trauma. *Hospital and Community Psychiatry* 1989; 40(1).

Sharan P et al. Preliminary report of psychiatric disorders in survivors of a severe earthquake. *American Journal of Psychiatry* 1996;153:4.

Tyhurst JS. Psychological and social aspects of civilian disaster. *Canadian Medical Association Journal* 1957;76:383-393.

Wilson JS, Keane TM (eds.). *Assessing psychological trauma and PTSD*. New York: The Guilford Press; 1997.

Applied and operational guidelines for assisting post-disaster survivors

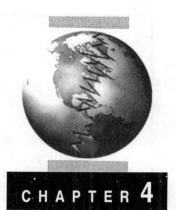

CHAPTER 4

- EDUCATION
- CONSULTATION
- OUTREACH
- CRISIS COUNSELING

■ TRAINING MODULE

Module 4:

Introduces post-disaster intervention programs and applied and operational guidelines.

■ WHY HAVE THIS MODULE?

To review the purpose, scope, and application of post-disaster assistance guidelines.

■ CONTENT

Similarities and differences vis-à-vis other types of mental health intervention programs.

- Special characteristics of post-disaster assistance
- Consultation
- Education
- Outreach
- Crisis Counseling

◼◼◼ LEARNING OBJECTIVES

After participating in Module 4 the students will:

Be able to identify existing outreach methodologies available to disaster mental health workers and plan post-disaster therapeutic interventions.

* Outreach
* Education
* Consultation
* Crisis counseling and support assistance

Referral to specialized programs

* Health
* Mental health
* Substance abuse
* Rehabilitation

◼◼◼ CONTENT SUMMARY

This module presents the basic mental health post-disaster interventions, which include the following:

OUTREACH: This procedure is designed to find and assist survivors in expressing and understanding disaster-caused stress and grief reactions.
CRISIS COUNSELING: This procedure uses techniques that assist the survivor to return to normal functioning. A small number of survivors will have to be referred for professional assistance from a specialist (e.g., children, elderly persons, substance abusers).
EDUCATION: This method of informing the public, agency workers, and mental health professionals can be done through the print media, television, and radio.
CONSULTATION: Can be used by experienced workers who will assist the public and private agencies deployed to develop emergency programs.

Training in outreach and crisis counseling is the most operationally driven type of training and will necessitate practical role-playing, as well as ongoing supervision once the workers begin to interact with survivors. Intervention approaches after a disaster need to be adapted according to (1) the characteristics of survivors and (2) the time that has elapsed after the disaster. Continuous awareness of the importance of cultural factors in counseling methods should be a strong focus of the training.

■■■■ TEACHING RESOURCES

Suggestions for using the teaching resources in this module: Teaching aids should be selected from the following pages based on the knowledge, functions, and responsibilities of the student population.

a. Post-disaster education: A list of key educational opportunities is presented for review. Others available in the affected community may be added.

b. Post-disaster consultation: A list of issues is presented to highlight the nature and objectives of the consultative process.

c. Educational consultancy on mental health aspects of disaster assistance: Presents the categories that should be considered when planning consulting activities.

d. Crisis theory and applied principles: A list of activities is presented to highlight the different aspects of intervention.

e. Planning a post-disaster intervention: Summarizes how the activities change over time and identifies elements found in all programs.

f. Several sheets define, describe, and operationalize the process of intervention.

Note to Trainer: The following pages are ready to be used as transparencies, slides, or handouts.

From disaster experiences to disaster assistance, a template for a post-disaster program is formed.

1. Sequence of human behavior

2. Outreach crisis intervention

3. Planning and mobilizing counseling intervention

4. Consultation

5. Education

6. Program for "special" situations

7. "Burn-out" syndrome among caretakers

8. Utilization of primary care workers

9. Cross-cultural issues in disaster assistance

10. Utilization of the private sector in disaster programs

POST-DISASTER EDUCATION

1. Communicate post-disaster advise and guidance via the mass media—TV, radio, newspaper—throughout each post-disaster phase.

2. Disseminate educational material to inform the population of "normal reactions in an abnormal situation."

3. Be prepared and accessible to media professionals to respond to their questions.

4. Be prepared to participate with lay groups to inform them about post-disaster reactions.

5. Write, print, and disseminate pamphlets, documents, cartoons, etc. with advice and guidance for survivors.

Stuhlmiller CM. *Rescuers of Cypress: Learning from disaster.* New York: Peter Lang; 1996.

Terr L. Childhood traumas: an outline and overview. *American Journal of Psychiatry* 1991; 148:10-20.

Tierney KJ, Baisden B. *Crisis intervention programs for disaster victims: a source book and manual for smaller communities.* Washington, D.C.: Government Printing Office; 1979. (DHHS Publication No. (ADM) 90-675).

Wolf ME, Mosnaim AD (eds.). Posttraumatic stress disorder: etiology, phenomenology, and treatment. Washington, D.C.: American Psychiatric Press; 1990.

Populations with special needs

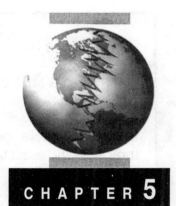

CHAPTER **5**

■ **TRAINING MODULE**

Module 5:

Identifies special populations at risk after a disaster and their specific assistance needs

■ **WHY HAVE THIS MODULE?**

To categorize the specific needs identified after a disaster and present effective types of post-disaster intervention

■ **CONTENT**

• Characteristics of different populations and their needs

• Children

• Elderly populations

• Persons with mental illness

• Persons with HIV/AIDS

• Persons with substance abuse problems

• Post-disaster caregivers and workers

▉ LEARNING OBJECTIVES:

After participating in Module 6 the student will be able to:

• Identify and describe the characteristic reactions of special populations affected by a disaster.
• Describe the interventions needed to assist populations at risk.

   a. Children
   b. Elderly populations
   c. Persons with mental illness
   d. Persons with HIV/AIDS
   e. Persons with substance abuse problems
   f. Post-disaster caregivers and workers

▉ SPECIAL RISK GROUPS

▉ CONTENT SUMMARY

There are many feelings and reactions that people share in common response to the direct and indirect effects of a disaster. However, special attention should be planned for persons in certain age groups and or those handicapped by certain social circumstances or by physical or emotional disabilities. This module describes some of these groups. It begins with a review of some of the thoughts, feelings, and behaviors common to all at-risk populations that experience a disaster.

▉ COMMON REACTIONS

1. Basic survival behavior
2. Increased stress due to loss of loved ones or loss of prized possessions
3. Separation anxiety, also expressed as fear for safety of significant others (predominant in children)
4. Regressive behaviors, e.g., reappearance of bed-wetting among children
5. Relocation anxieties and depression
6. Need to talk about experiences during the disaster
7. Wish to be part of the community and its rehabilitation efforts

▉ SPECIAL NEEDS GROUPS

The responses and needs of "special" populations affected by a disaster vary according to the characteristics of these populations—for example, developmental stage in children or differing degrees of capacity to cope in individuals suffering from mental illness. Trainers should develop additional presentations on these populations, augmented by teaching resources and group exercises that highlight their specific needs and the counseling modalities to assist them.

Members of special needs groups are among those most frequently encountered by workers providing counseling services in disaster areas. Some communities will have a unique or unusual composition, with the subgroups identified below.

1. Age groups
2. Socioeconomic classes
3. Cultural and racial groups
4. Persons institutionalized in acute care, general, and mental hospitals, and those in convalescent and correctional facilities
5. Survivors manifesting different intensities of emotional crisis
6. Survivors requiring emergency medical care
7. Human service and disaster relief workers

Age Groups

Each age period is accompanied by special problems which must be dealt with in everyday living. Some age groups, however, appear to be vulnerable in unique ways to the stresses of disaster. Research indicates that, in disaster situations, younger children and older adults are subject to significantly higher rates of fatalities and greater proportions of emotional and physical traumata when compared with the general population. Adolescents as a group are susceptible to unique and possible long-range effects of disaster as a result of the disruption of their peer group activities and a lack of access to full adult responsibilities in community rehabilitation efforts.

The following module subcomponents should be reproduced and distributed to workers who need specialized training to meet the needs of these population groups. To use the material on children, it is necessary to have a basic knowledge of child psychology. Again, the cultural characteristics of the community in which the disaster has occurred should be explored and used to adapt the generic material that follows. Exercises, vignettes, or videos should also reflect the culture of the community. For the subcomponent on persons with mental illness, medical help/consultation will be necessary. For the subcomponent on post-disaster caregivers and workers, it should be borne in mind that many workers are also survivors and may have experienced severe losses themselves. In addition to emergency workers, other professionals (such as teachers, policemen, hospital workers, mortuary staff) need to be considered both as workers and survivors).

CHILDREN

◼◼◼ CONTENT SUMMARY

The effects of a disaster on a child population produce a variety of reactions that are specific for each survivor, depending on a group of variables. Hence, the interplay of the type, extent, and proximity of the impact on a child within a family living in a geographical area has to be conceptualized based on knowledge of child psychology and disaster experiences. Of all these variables, the quality of attention given to the child's subsequent needs and the parental reactions emerge as particularly significant.

Problems will vary depending upon the phase of the post-disaster period. Some problems may appear weeks or months later. Crisis workers should alert the parents to the potential for their occurrence and the phase in which they may appear. In general, children of all ages will show a combination of these symptoms: sleep disturbances, persistent fears about recurring weather events or future disasters, and loss of interest in daily activities, especially school.

Published descriptions of clinical and behavioral manifestations of children's reactions to traumatic events focus on biological, psychological, interpersonal, and social perspectives. Documented observations of post-traumatic reactions in children suffer from the lack of consensus among researchers about data-gathering, which adds to the difficulty of developing a comprehensive frame of reference.

Because the conceptualization of children's reactions is influenced by (1) the event itself, (2) the degree of disorganization within the family, (3) the impact on social structures, and (4) the attention given to the child's subsequent needs, it is difficult to design materials which identify and correlate all the factors that affect the child's behavior. The importance of parental response to children's level of distress has been identified as a powerful influence. The need to plan, develop, and offer assistance to the victims of traumatic events is prompting further study of programs to prevent pathological effects on the child's health and negative emotional consequences.

The emerging knowledge about the psychosocial processes that serve the function of adaptation at different levels of child development is filling a need for further knowledge in disaster planning. Experiences are accumulating and being shared, allowing professionals to develop tentative methods of intervention. Questions about how to intervene with children after a disaster raise a classic dilemma in crisis counseling. It is necessary to apply a consistent model to organize the information obtained, develop a child crisis theory, and select the appropriate intervention approach. A useful conceptual approach in this situation can be obtained by focusing on the stressful event in which the child finds him/herself and adopting a framework of understanding the child as an evolving interacting organism within a bio-psycho-socio-cultural environment.

There is a relationship between the approaches through which problems are defined and the intervention that is chosen and then translated into action. Post-disaster problem definition reflects inferences and assumptions about the causes of the problem. In the case of post-traumatic stress reactions in children, the reactive-adaptive behavior that can be observed following the impact of a disaster is related to (1) the child's stage of development; (2) the child's sex and ethnicity and the economic status of the family; (3) the child's usual coping defense style; (4) the intensity of the stressor; (5) availability and appropriate "fit" between the child's needs and support systems; (6) the extent of dislocation; and (7) availability of relief and community disaster assistance resources. Collecting specific data about the survivor and organizing the data to pinpoint the problems produced by the situation in which the child finds him/herself provides guidance for the development of appropriate interventions. The way the data gets organized, all the unique characteristics that identify the survivor, the hypothetical interaction among all the factors and how they affect the child's capacity to cope are based on the assumptions chosen by the crisis counselor.

Several areas of theoretical knowledge will be highlighted because they are crucial to the understanding of behavior in post-disaster experiences and are key for intervention programs.

■ RELATIONSHIP BETWEEN CHILDREN'S DEVELOPMENTAL STAGES AND POST-DISASTER REACTIONS

As children grow and pass through the various developmental stages, changes take place in several psychobiological systems. Depending on the age of the child traumatized by the event, the intervention should be designed based on knowledge about the developmental stage of different systems: somatic, psychological, social, and behavioral. There is a relationship between the level achieved in these systems and the ability to deal with the stressful events following the disaster. Adaptive processes can be understood as strategies, approaches, or efforts that promote action whose objective is to modify the impact of the stimuli unleashed by the stressor and so tolerate, correct, modify, or diminish the effects on the organism and prevent reactive disorganization within the psychophysiological human system. These adaptive skills and their effects on the vulnerable organism of the child will be manifested in a variety of behavior patterns. The interpretation of these manifestations of the child's adaptation mechanism, the social expectations toward him within the disorganized human environment, and the social and family conflicts that generally emerge in a crisis situation will determine the level of coping and adaptation, which, in turn, will influence the methods of assistance and intervention chosen. For instance, the reactions to an earthquake of a one-year-old child, who processes stimuli and information through an evolving cognitive system, will be different from those of an older child, who will use a symbolic-linguistic mode of information processing.

■ PSYCHIC TRAUMA AND DEVELOPMENTAL EXPRESSIONS OF MOURNING AFTER A DISASTER

An important body of knowledge is beginning to reveal the processes available to children during traumatic events that involve loss. For a child, the death or psychological unavailability of a nurturant person is not only a traumatic event, but it also constitutes a very serious developmental interference. As the child advances through the growth of multiple systems, mastering the various psychological and emotional tasks needed to achieve maturity, a stimulating interaction with his/her love objects is essential. Depending on their stage of development and cognitive/ affective capacities, children will manifest differing behavior patterns expressive of disrupted organization, regressive functions, infantile emotional manifestation and patterns of cognitive functions, which incorporate the developed level of their subunits (reality thinking, abstract reasoning, causality).

In post-disaster experiences, besides the stage of development, the dynamic implications of loss and their interaction with reactive processes to the trauma set up by the disaster must be considered. All disasters are dramatic events that are accompanied by visual and auditory experiences that are incomprehensible at the moment of occurrence. Hearing the preliminary sounds of an earthquake, watching the earth open up, seeing buildings collapse all produce anxiety reactions of different levels of intensity. These are concrete, frightening events that are mentally recorded and will be internal traumatic repetitive stimuli to several infantile emotions. When these are accompanied by subsequent loss of a parent, it is difficult to sort out whether the child's reactions are indications of psychic trauma or early signs of mourning. In addition to differential needs, reactions accompanying loss should be incorporated into the evaluation and intervention guidelines.

■ RISK FACTORS IN POST-TRAUMATIC CRISIS RESOLUTION

The child's level of psychobiological function is related to the vulnerability of the child's developmental stage, biological health, and personality strength. It needs to be ascertained whether the child is showing high anxiety, depression, withdrawal, regression, disturbance of sleep and eating functions in order to measure the manifestation of disorganized psychobiological factors. To be able to measure these signals, the professional must investigate the following:

1. The psychosocial maturity or immaturity of the child;
2. The social expectations of performance behavior as judged by the child, his/her family, and others living with them;
3. Continued environmental post-disaster stress, both in social and physical accommodations, throughout the period of transition;
4. Accidental crisis events occurring in the child's life, either before or after the stressor event;
5. Social settings as post-disaster stressors.

The setting in which the child is located is an important variable that will affect the choice of psychological intervention. This statement is based on the realistic, practical experience of housing victims in crowded sheltered settings. The rapid turnover of large numbers of victims in and out of the shelter and the small number of trained staff who remain with the same family for extended periods of time influence the type of intervention. What might be the best type of intervention within the specific setting, given the available resources?

■ INTERVENTION PROGRAM FOR CHILDREN—CRISIS INTERVENTION

Development and implementation of mental health services to help children suffering from the psychological consequences of a disaster have to be designed taking account the context, post-disaster timeframe, and characteristics of the identified population. Although children's responses may differ from event to event, it is possible to develop broad guidelines for the design and execution of post-disaster psychological services. The elements that enter into the design of a plan will focus only on the child population. It is assumed that a complex overall mental health program with different multilevel services is already in place; the child mental health program will be embedded and coordinated with the other services so as to delivery psychological aid effectively to all victims. The objective of the program will be the implementation of mental health intervention services for children affected by a disaster or catastrophic event. This is done with the understanding that there are many other types of services needed in such situations—for example, feeding, housing, medical services, and recreational activities.

■ DIRECT MENTAL HEALTH SERVICES—EARLY PHASE

The mental health intervention program can be organized along two major lines of professional activity. The first is direct face-to-face intervention with families housed in emergency shelters. Crisis counselors who start working directly with the families and the relocation centers will be available to offer psychological help to a gathered group of families in need. Guided by their knowledge of the time phases and the sequential manifestation of crisis phenomenology, the workers can identify and organize a number of approaches to help children and their families through the phases of crisis, coping, and adaptation. As these families move through their evolving situation of emergency housing and changing human environments, they will exhibit different behaviors and express different needs in different phases of crisis resolution. The crisis counselor will develop interventive procedures to meet the objective of returning the family and the children to a functional level of adaptation. As mentioned before, the objective of crisis counseling is successful use of techniques that (1) restore the capacity of children to function by assisting them in handling the stressful situation in which they find themselves; and (2) assist the family in reorganizing its world through social support and guidance from the crisis counselor. This can be accomplished through collaboration and referral by the counselor to other support and care-giving emergency assistance groups, with all the family welfare agencies helping the children and their caregivers.

■ THERAPEUTIC CRISIS INTERVENTION FOR FAMILIES

Crisis intervention encompasses all the activities by which the worker/counselor seeks to relieve the distress of the child and assist the family through counseling. It encompasses all helping activities based on communication, which is primarily, though not necessarily, verbal interaction. Many of the families display a sense of hopelessness and demoralization. All forms of counseling use certain approaches to combat and control this painful effect. Demoralized families show behavior that reflects the feeling of being unable to cope with the multiple tasks that families have when taking care of children and that others expect them to handle well. These families' sense of self can vary widely after a disaster. The signs of demoralization in a family might include the following:

1. They express feelings of diminished self-confidence and have difficulty recognizing their ability to handle the children's and their own needs.
2. They believe that failure will be the outcome of their decisions and actions, and they appear to be struggling with feelings of guilt and shame as part of the adaptive regression.
3. The family feels alienated, depressed, and isolated, as if they had been singled out for the worst outcome.
4. The family is enmeshed in a sense of increased dependency on agency workers who may have difficulty in understanding both the confused intrafamilial reactive feelings and the family value systems based on traditional ethnic ways of behaving in a novel situation.

■ TECHNIQUES FOR HELPING FAMILIES ACROSS THE DEVELOPMENTAL PHASES OF CRISIS RESOLUTION FOR FAMILIES

Several techniques are available to the counselor who is interested in intervening during the sequential phases of crisis manifested by families and children traumatized by a disaster. These initial techniques can be grouped under the heading of "auxiliary first aid techniques." These early approaches are directed initially toward restoring family functions and helping the family adapt to the early transition experience; they can also be instrumental in reintegrating and returning the total family system to balance. Intervention procedures are related to helping the family assess, solve problems, and make decisions day by day as they move through the emergency situation, the reconstruction phase, and, finally, return to a more permanent living situation. These approaches are defined as any active interaction between the counselor and the family that tends to supplement, complement, reinforce, and promote family systems mechanisms in the new setting. By restoring the family's functions and adaptive strategies, the child is assisted in functioning more effectively.

The following is an example of this approach:

A family composed of a mother (36 years old) and father (41 years old) with two children (8 and 12 years old), were found in one of the shelters. A major avalanche had buried their neighborhood a few hours after they had climbed to safety on a nearby hill. They had to spend six to eight hours in the cold night air before being rescued by emergency workers, who brought them to the shelter, where they were fed and offered some cots and blankets. The counselor who met with them observed that the mother was crying and appeared somewhat dazed and depressed, while the father was trying to actively organize the family activities and cheer everyone up. The children seemed to adapt to the new surroundings, and although their faces expressed tension, they did not appear to show gross behavior disturbances. Following a preliminary evaluation of the situation, it was obvious that the most expressive disturbance of feelings was manifested by the mother. A short evaluation proved that she had been unable to relax, her thinking was depressed, and she felt hopeless and helpless. The father, on the other hand, appeared to deny the reality of the situation and tried to encourage the family with false and unrealistic hopes. After a few days, the children began to lose their ability to cope, became more demanding and restless, had difficulty in eating and sleeping, and did not want to separate from the mother to go out onto the playground that had been organized for children in the shelter.

The intervention was designed to complement the mother's ability to feel more competent and reinforce the father's sense of "being in charge" through a realistic approach so that he would not have to deny and distort reality to regain his composure. The total family was helped to express some of their sadness and feeling of disorientation through the provision of knowledge, daily news, and explanations about what was going to happen in the present and in the next few days. The children were able to meet in small groups with other children, where they shared their memories about the event and were offered the possibility of expressing some of their fantasies through drawings so as to promote a sense of mastery over their feelings. The parents were asked to assist in the housekeeping duties of the shelter and to participate in organized adult activities.

The process described above provides a prototypical example of the range of procedures (behavior, actions, speech, types of meetings, face-to-face interactions) through which intervention occurs and is adapted to the situation encountered. The child and his family in the early stages of relocation will express through behavior the manifestations of the crisis and the methods of coping they are using. The resources available to the counselor will influence the procedures that can be used, the time that can be spent with the family and the activities that are available in the relocation center. The crisis counseling approach varies because different combinations of factors come into play, depending on the extent of community disruption and the availability of resources. But the objective remains clear: to restore the adaptive system of the family, which, in turn, will help the children control the regressive behaviors seen in all traumatized children.

Crisis counseling for children must be based on the ability to conceptualize and understand the crisis manifestations and the levels of infantile dysfunction during the various stages of post-disaster crisis resolution.

■ STEPS AND GUIDELINES FOR CRISIS INTERVENTION FOR FAMILIES

The crisis counselor establishes a relationship with the family and the child by explaining and educating the family about the psychological processes that occur in the wake of a disaster. The intervention objectives are set by (1) obtaining the information needed to plan the approach; (2) establishing credibility and gaining the family's confidence; (3) describing the intervention plan; and (4) eliciting the family's cooperation in the plan. From all this data-gathering, the crisis counselor arrives at a tentative formulation of the problem and/or the plan of action. The objectives are to alleviate the emotional distress in the family and the cognitive disorganization in the child as a first strategy.

The following key principles guide the sequential steps of intervention:

* Crisis counselors should assume that families are potentially capable of handling their own problems after being helped to recognize the areas of distress and redirect their behavior towards exploring new solutions.
* Counselors should allow the family to develop initial dependency so that the family can "borrow" confidence from the counselor and, at the same time, offer it to their children. This stage should be short-lived; long-term dependency should be discouraged.
* Counselors should generally be cautious about giving advice, although this does not preclude their informing the family about all relevant matters on which they are ignorant or misinformed. Such information will help the family solve its own problems.
* Whenever possible, depending on the age of the child, the counselor should seek to help the child understand the linkages between feelings and behavior. This may help the family understand the feelings and thoughts that signal actual progression toward crisis resolution; it will also allow the family to make sense of and put into perspective feelings that are disturbing, which will enhance their sense of mastery and control.
* Emotions that are seen in the initial post-trauma phases include sadness, fear, and anger. These are manifested in many forms and with a wide range of intensity. The counselor should accept these emotions as expressions of the pain the families have suffered and support their perspective of the event. Assistance in achieving resignation and acceptance of the reality of the situation in which they find themselves is part of the process of post-disaster grieving.

Some families temporarily become cognitively and emotionally disorganized. The intervention needs to be directed toward remedying this disorganization, as it interferes with parenting tasks. Steps should be taken to increase parents' competence and maintain their awareness that the situation generated by the disaster will demand increased individual mobilization of all their parenting skills to help their children adapt to an environment of trauma. The counselor should offer support and encouragement to strengthen the parents' conscious awareness of appropriate social reactions in light of what is happening. This clarification is encouraging and useful for reinforcing natural parental behavior. Continued cognitive disorganization will affect the family's ability to deal with their problems and their children's problems. One of the primary aims in such cases is to help the family diminish the effects of the disorganization and reinforce their cognitive mastery by offering counseling assistance that is useful according to their specific conditions. By helping the family to diminish their sense of helplessness, their indecisive or regressive behavior, and their belief that they lack coping skills, the counselor enables the family to rebuild itself more rapidly and begin to assume responsibility for child care. By guiding families and assisting them in problem- solving and in dealing with the children directly when the children are showing signs of emotional disturbance, the counselor helps the family to pull together and continue to move forward along the crisis resolution pathway.

■ STRATEGIES FOR INTERVENTION FOR FAMILIES

Setting priorities for action and selecting displaced families to assist in the first few days following a disaster is a difficult triage process. As soon as families are identified, they need help to regain a sense of orientation, reinforce reality, and develop support and trust. Ascertaining families' needs for the type of resources that can be obtained and provided by other agencies is the responsibility of the crisis worker.

A wide array of resources are available to families through emergency programs, but they must be organized to meet their specific needs. Many of those needs are concrete, but others are psychological. The crisis worker can mobilize appropriate help by observing the way staff from other agencies behave or approach the family. This requires a special technique that allows the worker to elicit directly and personally from the family, in their own communication style, what they perceive as immediate needs, interpret those needs within the context of the available programs, and then collaborate with other agencies in mobilizing the resources so that the family and the children feel assisted, less helpless, less hopeless and destitute.

■ EARLY AND LATE AFTERMATH PHASES FOR FAMILIES

As families are relocated from emergency shelters to temporary lodgings or back to their own homes—which may be damaged but safe—a new stage of crisis emerges, manifested by expressions of increased grieving and bereavement. The crisis worker needs to develop a combination of activities that include outreach in order to follow relocated families and monitor the children's progression toward a return of function. The worker should assess the family's level of adaptation, and if the assessment does not reveal further decompensation, the worker can let the family know that he/she is available if needed. If the family notices a psychological problem or wishes to further utilize community resources, they can recontact the emergency assistance team.

It is during this sequence of post-disaster phases that children's level of development and previous experience play the greatest role in their coping mechanisms and degree of adaptation. Young children appear to rely heavily on denial as a means of accommodating the traumatic event. As children develop the ability to express their ideas, they can talk more often about frightening episodes, share experiences, reproduce distressing visual impressions in drawings, and express conflicts through repetitive play. Older children appear to respond to explicit, directive, and encouraging discussion with crisis counselors.

The same strategies that were useful in the shelters—approaching daily activities through an accurate cognitive appraisal of the situation, enhancing the family's knowledge about their surroundings so that they can understand both their own emotions and external events—appear to aid families during subsequent stages and increase their adaptive capacity, diminishing the level of depression and anxiety. If appropriate and feasible, group intervention, with parents or teachers getting together with children to discuss how they are responding to stress and what is expected as natural, healthy crisis resolution behavior, also appears to enhance adaptation.

The method of bringing parents and children together in groups is helpful because the children's problems tend to get overlooked as family members are overwhelmed not only by their own personal feelings but by the enormity of the task of reconstructing their concrete world, which takes priority. The crisis counselor's function is to provide support, offer him/herself as someone to whom the parents can come in case of difficulties, clarify the child's behavior, and suggest methods of controlling it. Often, too, the counselor will need to mobilize other social agencies, including the school, to help families who are having difficulty in adapting to their new setting and who are disrupted or have difficulty in coping with the ordinary demands of family life. At times, working with the school may be essential to provide a child with additional assistance, and contact with other adults may be helpful to the family. To enable parents to use other social and practical resources in the community is part of educating them to the fact that they may need assistance to carry out their duties for a short time, without suggesting that agencies take over their parental role. Every decision must be theirs, and it is they who must initiate every change in the sequence of life activities that will lead them to a recovery of their family dynamic balance.

▬▬ TEACHING RESOURCES

▮ CHILDREN

a. Reactive Phase
A list of reactions by age is presented to highlight the different reactions that occur in children at different developmental stages.
b. Several models of intervention for families and children are described.

The following pages are ready for use as transparencies, slides, or handouts.

IMPACT OF STRESSORS

Key variables that influence children's reactions/ consequences:

• Speed of onset

• Duration of the trauma

• Potential for recurrence

• Degree of life threat

• Degree of exposure to death, dying, and destruction

• Proportion of the family affected

• Role of the caregiver in the trauma

• Degree of displacement in home continuity

• Separation from nuclear family

• Rekindling of childhood anxieties

• Communicated anxiety between parents and children

• Cultural expectations

Smith, W. [...] [...] Organ [...] and Application [...] New York, [...] Press, 198[...]

Lin, J. Childhood syndrome, its quality and [...] of use [...] American [...]: [...] [...] 19[...] [...]:51–60.

Black, M. J.; Weber, H. Cover and culture program: building a better economy and care manual for small [...] economics, Washington, D.C.: [...] public Publications [...] 6 [...] 1986 [...] Publication No. [...] 1989–83].

Van der Meulen, A. P. van, [...] Performance improvement can employ maximum care [...]: [...] training. Washington [...] Management Association, [...] 66 pp.

PSYCHIC TRAUMA PRODUCED BY A CATASTROPHIC EVENT

Key Issues

- The child's reactions will vary according to his/her stage of cognitive, affective, and sociobehavioral development.

- The reactive phenomena observed after a catastrophic event represent bio-psycho-social systems reactions and early efforts to cope with the disorganization of these systems.

  a) Need to re-establish capacity to regulate intense affect

  b) Need to formulate cognitive appraisal of initial event and subsequent evolving experiences.

  c) Need to restore bodily integrity

- Family and societal behavior toward a child is a powerful influence that can enhance or impede the trauma resolution process. The child's reliance on the family for cognitive guidance and socioemotional support is influenced by the child's stage of psychosexual development and pre-existent psychopathology.

- A mourning process accompanies all catastrophic psychic trauma due to loss of body configuration (if injured), interpersonal bonds (quantity/quality), worldview and familiarity, expectations and trust.

- Reactive depression as a clinical syndrome needs to be differentiated from the expression of psychic trauma and an effective/ineffective mourning outcome.

IMPACT OF CATASTROPHIC EVENTS

Direct impact on child

Body trauma - pain, autonomic arousal, increased tension, loss of function
Sensory changes - visual, auditory, olfactory
Emotional expressions - fear, distress, anxiety
Cognition changes - language, communication.

Indirect impact on child

Traumatic reactions of parents, siblings, friends, and extended family
Disorganization of social systems - school, church, father's/mother's employment, housing

REACTIVE PHASE RESPONSES OF CHILDREN TO A CATASTROPHIC EVENT

Preschool Child

Somatic systems
- Muscular immobilization, hyper-activity
- Temper tantrums, slow movements, not goal-directed
- Disorganization of acquired body functions
- Autonomic nervous system signs, vomiting, crying
- Sleeping/eating disturbances, pale skin, hyperventilation
- Wide pupil stare, startle reactions

Affective system
- Constricted/flat affect
- Detachment
- Rage/aggressive responses
- Fear/worry
- Anxious/suspicious

Cognitive system
- Recurrent memories, thoughts, fantasies of event
- Disturbed dream content
- Decrease of acquired performance, language
- Visual-spatial, concentration
- Distorted description of visual phenomena

Social behavior system
- Avoidance, dependence, passive/intense, energetic/impulsive
- Partial loss of toilet training
- Increased autoerotic activity
- Abrupt, destructive play

REACTIVE PHASE RESPONSES OF CHILDREN TO A CATASTROPHIC EVENT (continued)

School Age Child

Somatic systems
- Energy level affected
- Movements slow, low-intensity, or rapid, frenetic, impulsive
- Autonomic disorganization; appetite/sleep/ elimination

Affective system
- Lability of affect; anxious, sad, giggly, "nervous"
- Cautious; afraid to take chances or return to familiar places
- Increased fear of competition, of losing, of getting lost
- Increased dependency/decreased independence feelings
- Increased susceptibility of emotional reactions to sensory reminders of the traumatic event
- Initial process of mourning and reactions to loss

Cognitive system
- Constriction and hypervigilant alertness
- Intellectual functions affected; dull, obtuse
- Obsessive rumination and increased distractibility affecting memory loss
- Decreased associations leading to spontaneous reminder of event characteristics
- Increased fantasizing about how they could have changed events, controlled outcome of the incident
- Appearance of learning problems

Social behavior system
- Obsessive-compulsive expressive play, talk, curiosity about event and its consequences
- Inconsistent, capricious reactions to parents
- Argumentative and disobedient
- Poor impulse control
- Difficulty returning to routines
- Some loss of habits, customs, skills

VARIABLES THAT INFLUENCE POST-DISASTER REACTIONS IN CHILDREN

1. Serious disruption of developmental processes will produce disorganization in all psychological expressions.

2. Special significance of the event and post-disaster experiences will be related to the stage of development.

3. The quality of family relations will affect the expression of mourning manifestations.

4. The intensity of the physical and psychological trauma will influence the mourning process and lengthen the duration of the post-disaster reactions.

5. Special circumstances surrounding the child's life before the disaster (divorce, new school, surgery, immigration) should be taken into account in assessing the child.

6. The reactions to these events by important adults in the child's life should also be considered.

7. For a child who has lost his/her family, the multiple changes in the environment following the disaster are other important variables.

8. Plasticity and resiliency as protective factors should be evaluated during intervention.

VARIABLES ASSISTING IN THE RECOVERY OF FAMILIES

1. Developing structures and networks
2. Establishing reliable schedules
3. Choosing activities that enhance self-esteem, such as volunteer activities
4. Continued strengthening of social contacts
5. Becoming involved in group activities
6. Attending to material/personal needs
7. Recognizing that relationships and attachments act as regulators and modulators of emotions and cognitive systems organization, which influence patterns of relationships
8. Identifying risk factors - (action/interaction - individual - environment)
9. Learning or asking advice about children's reactions at home and in school
10. Using all available help and resources

Certain families may be especially vulnerable and can be identified in this process:

- Families with pre-existing marital or functional problems
- Deprived multiproblem families for whom this disaster may prove to be the "last straw"
- Families who are dislocated into systems that cannot or do not support them
- Families who have suffered overwhelming loss, trauma, and/or separation
- Families severely affected by survivor guilt
- Families who have split, disintegrated, or decompensated following the disaster

OBJECTIVES OF INTERVENTION

1. To help the child develop an internal sense of perspective so that he/she will be able to organize his/her own environment.

2. To assist the recuperative process of sharing painful emotions provoked by the stressor events, which will help the child (according to his/her age) put events into perspective.

3. To help the child reach out to both his/her family members and the professionals on the emergency teams in order to use the resources that are available to develop a sense of comfort, security, and affection.

INTERVENTION STRATEGIES TO ADDRESS SECONDARY STRESSES

1. Monitor secondary stresses for the child and family

2. Assist the child in identifying sources of secondary stress

3. Address emotional responses

4. Address interference with developmental opportunities

5. Enhance coping skills

TREATMENT OF REACTIVITY TO TRAUMATIC REMINDERS

1. Identification of traumatic reminders

2. Increase child's understanding of the traumatic reference

3. Assistance with cognitive discrimination

4. Increase tolerance for expectable reactivity

5. Address missed developmental opportunities due to traumatic avoidance

Current intervention practice for children includes three main points (long term):

- An opportunity for exposure to a disaster's frightening elements in a non-threatening atmosphere. Activities such as drawing pictures, sharing stories, and playing "hurricane games" let children relive the hurricane and deal with it.

- The development of skills to cope with issues that remain difficult, such as property losses and adjustment to new surroundings.

- Access to supportive social relationships when a disaster has affected the child's loved ones' ability to cope.

POST-DISASTER MENTAL HEALTH ASSISTANCE MODEL FOR CHILDREN (LONG TERM)

- An individual diagnostic and treatment service should be available for children and their families who identify themselves as in need of help and/or who are referred for psychological assistance.

- Special consultation services for social agencies that work in the post-disaster program. Direct links between the psychological teams and the agencies should be cultivated. Special problem cases should be referred for discussion and problem-solving to assist the social agencies in obtaining resources for the family and the child.

- A program of regular group discussions with the professionals who work with children should be organized. The aim is to help these professionals deal with their current problems and increase their therapeutic, supportive, and healing skills. Because assisting children who are orphaned or separated from their parents following a disaster is such a new component of social welfare systems, professionals need regular help and support in their dealings with the children and in their contacts with relatives.

- Consultation to schools should be offered for long-term follow-up of traumatized children.

COUNSELING TRAUMATIZED CHILDREN
A COUNSELING
MODEL (LONG TERM)

Relationship-building and information-gathering regarding the trauma

The mental health worker describes the purpose and process for assisting children who have been traumatized. He/she proceeds to gather details about the trauma from the family and child.

Assessment of the child and the child's family

The mental health worker gathers information regarding the family structure and the child's experience in the disaster, previous traumatic experiences, addictions patterns, and the presence of consequences or symptoms of post-traumatic stress reactions.

Trauma interview

The mental health worker facilitates the child's telling of the traumatic experience through drawings or role-playing, encouraging attention to specific details, including sights, sounds, smells, and accountability for the event.

Identification of post-disaster issues

The mental health worker identifies issues that need to be addressed with the child, such as difficulty coping with nightmares, physiologic reactivity, or impulse control.

Issues are also identified for the family, including management of their own and their child's post-trauma consequences and parenting and communication skills

Post-disaster intervention methods

Short-term play therapy, activity therapy, family therapy, group therapy are provided, based on the age of the child and the needs of the family post-disaster.

Consultations are held with other service providers, including the school system, social services, foster parents, etc.

Relapse Prevention

The intervention goal is for the child and family to have the skills to cope with post-trauma consequences and situations.

The return of some post-disaster problems is expected and viewed as normal. The child and family identify situations in which the consequences of trauma might get worse.

The family is encouraged to return to counseling if necessary.

■ GROUP WORK/EXERCISES

- After viewing the *Children and Trauma* video (CMHS-ESDRB) or a similar video, identify the intervention techniques.
- Write a post-disaster script for role-play:
  a. a family with two children aged 6 and 12
  b. a group of children in a classroom
  c. an African-American family (or a family from another ethnic minority group) with three children
- Choose one "vignette" and role-play the intervention needed.
- Develop a list of possible signs of post-trauma stress in a boy whose parents were killed in a tornado.

ELDERLY POPULATIONS

■■■■ CONTENT SUMMARY

Elderly populations have a number of characteristics and concerns that make them particularly vulnerable to the effects of disasters. They may respond in an ineffective manner due to slowing of motor and cognitive activity. Some older adults may experience further trauma if they are transferred to an unfamiliar, crowded setting. As a consequence of having lived for many years, elderly persons tend to experience multiple losses, including loss of important support systems. On the other hand, they may show resilience due to having successfully managed difficulties and coped with disappointments earlier in life. Workers should be alert to signs of depression among elderly survivors, since losses sustained from the disaster may add to previous losses and lead to depression.

Elderly populations have specific reactions and needs after a disaster. As with other subpopulations, workers need to consider many individual factors that distinguish one individual from another. However, generalizing about special subgroup needs helps to develop guidelines for the post-disaster program that will meet each group's needs.

Many older adults, especially those who are poor, immigrants, or unskilled, may lack resources, have declining physical capacity, and lose important support systems in the destroyed neighborhood. They may also have more difficulty in "navigating" the channels of the emergency system, or they may fear that they will lose their "independent" status if workers become aware of their diminished capacity.

Problems that may aggravate the problems of coping after a disaster for older persons include the following:

• Relocation with family members where privacy, personal space, and daily routines are a source of stress.
• Difficulty with sleeping schedules and relying on sleep medication
• Sense of disorganization or confusion due to losses of "cues" in daily activity.

Disaster workers may be able to relate better with elderly survivors by being aware of these characteristics. These examples serve as a reminder that the bio-psycho-social characteristics of specific populations must be considered when analyzing the risk factors that influence post-disaster coping capacity.

The training materials that follow will guide discussions and help identify other specific needs of this population and the corresponding interventions.

TRAUMA REACTIONS
OF OLDER ADULTS

▬▬ OVERVIEW

The reactions of older individuals to a trauma will be influenced not only by the impact of the catastrophe on their lives (what they saw, heard, felt, smelled, and so on), but by memories of crises in their past. This revisitation of past events is not simply a product of regression or trigger reactions. It is essentially a normal attempt to ground one's reactions in the familiar.

The following resources can be used to select a series of slides to high light key issues for the elderly.

TRAUMA REACTIONS

- Increased memories of past and friends or eras may color disaster effects

- May move in and out of disoriented state during first days in shelter

- May show increased dependence on current friends or family, refusing assistance from authorities

- Needs to integrate post-disaster changes into context of life after the disaster

- Disorientation as routine is interrupted; a sense of isolation both in terms of place and time after relocation

- Immediate response after shock, primarily fear, followed by anger and frustration if living conditions/setting is unfamiliar

- Physiological responses: sleep disturbances, appetite disturbances

- Sense of foreshortened future and retreat into past or fantasy for safety

REACTIONS TO TRAUMATIC EVENTS AMONG ELDERLY POPULATIONS

- Fear of mortality
- Need for permanence
- Wish to reconnect with past and with friends
- Regression
  — Generally temporary state
  — May be long-term regression of severe, chronic condition
  — May move in and out of regressed state during relocation
- Multiple Losses
  — Fear of relocation to unknown neighborhood
  — Fear of losing their dignity
  — Loss of hope for the future
  — Loss of cherished mementos
- Need to integrate loss into context of life
- Disorientation as routine is interrupted,
- Sense of isolation in terms of both place and time if too many relocations take place
- Use of denial as a normal defensive reaction to trauma
- Immediate fear response, followed by anger and frustration when unable to control a situation
- Physiological responses
  — sleep disturbances
  — appetite disturbances
  — muscle spasms

■ TO REINFORCE COPING STRATEGIES FOR ELDERS *

- **Rebuild and reaffirm attachments and relationships**: Relationships are the connection to life. Nurturing and physical closeness is needed. Let older persons identify those to whom they want to be attached; however, do not assume family relations are friendly.
- **Consider their concerns about safety:** The elderly need to know they have options in making a choice about their safety. Evacuation is a highly controversial issue in disaster. Older adults may be less safe in evacuations than if they remain in their homes (if this is feasible).
- **Talk about the tragedy:** Remember that older persons may be venting feelings about their lives, not about the immediate event. Do not attempt to prevent this venting, since validating past concerns is an important part of establishing trust in preparing to deal with current concerns.
- **Anticipate communication lapses:** In conversations, the elderly may go back and forth from the past to the present. Workers may be confused by an individual's discussion of past events or past relationships in terms of the present disaster experience. It is important to remember that the discussion may be entirely rational and logical from the perspective of the individual.
- **Understand that stress inhibits memory:** If an older person forgets a name, place, or portion of an event, the worker should take great precautions to avoid placing pressure on the elderly person to remember. In most cases, the elder will remember, but pressure inhibits memory.
- **Prepare for sporadic conversation:** Workers should be prepared for the elderly to talk sporadically about the disaster, spending small segments of time concentrating on particular aspects of the traumatic experience as a method of defense.
- **Be aware of cultural differences:** Workers should be aware that minority elders may have different cultural and traditional backgrounds. This will influence their worldview, especially the way they regard post-disaster services and public agencies. Services delivered to the dominant groups may not necessarily be suitable for every minority group.
- **Provide factual information:** Older adults want factual information, but may be able to absorb the facts only in limited quantity. Often, they ask to have information about the disaster repeated a number of times. Eventually they will integrate it and gain better control over their emotions about the event.

---

* Based on guidelines set out in documents published by various state, regional, and area agencies on aging in the United States.

- **Make short-term predictions**: The elderly should be given information on what will happen to them immediately after the disaster. Specific times and places for events should be made clear. It will help to delineate events on a calendar or clock so that the older person can more easily track the future. Workers should spend time addressing basic needs in a detailed way, such as who will help the older person, where the person will stay at night, where he/she will get clothes, and what property may be rescued.
- **Establish routines quickly:** It is best to reinitiate old routines if possible, since routines are considered an anchor in aging.
- **Reassure about normal reactions:** The worker should reassure the elderly that lapses of concentration, memory losses, physical ailments, and depression are normal reactions to tragedy and disaster.
- **Be supportive and build confidence:** The worker should strive to ensure that older persons maintain their self-confidence and dignity throughout all the post-disaster activities necessary to return them to their homes.

OLDER PERSONS AND THEIR RESPONSES *
Summary of Special Concerns

Sensory deprivation

Older persons' sense of smell, touch, vision, and hearing may be less acute than that of the general population. A hearing loss may cause an older person not to hear what is said in a noisy environment, or a diminished sense of smell may mean that he or she is more apt to eat spoiled food.

Delayed response syndrome

Older persons may not react to a situation as fast as younger persons. In disasters, this means that disaster assistance centers may need to be kept open longer if older persons have not appeared. It also means that older persons may not meet deadlines in applying for disaster assistance.

Generational differences

Depending on when individuals were born, they share differing values and expectations. This becomes important in service delivery, since what is acceptable to an 80-year-old person may not be acceptable to a person 65 years of age.

Chronic illness and medication use

Higher percentages of older persons have chronic conditions such as arthritis. This may prevent an older person from standing in line. Medications may cause confusion in an older person or a greater susceptibility to problems such as dehydration. These and other similar problems may increase their difficulties in obtaining post-disaster assistance.

Memory disorders

Environmental factors or chronic diseases may affect the ability of older persons to remember information or to act appropriately.

Transfer trauma

Frail older persons who are dislocated without use of proper procedures may suffer illness and even death.

Multiple loss effect

Many older persons have lost their spouses, income, homes, and/or physical capabilities. For some persons, these losses compound one other. Disasters sometimes represent a final blow, making recovery particularly difficult for older persons. One response may be an inappropriate attachment to specific items of property.

---

* Based on a guide published by the U.S. Administration on Aging, 1994.

(continued)

OLDER PERSONS AND THEIR RESPONSES*
Summary of Special Concerns
(continued)

Hyper/hypothermia vulnerability

Older persons are often much more susceptible to the effects of heat or cold. This becomes more critical in disasters, when furnaces and air conditioners may be unavailable or unserviceable.

Crime victimization

Con artists target older persons, particularly after a disaster. Other targeting by criminals may also develop. These issues need to be addressed in shelters and in housing arrangements.

Unfamiliarity with bureaucracy

Older persons often have not had any experience working through a bureaucratic system. This may be especially true for older widowed women whose spouses dealt with such matters.

Literacy

Many older persons have lower educational levels than the general population. This may cause difficulties in completion of applications or understanding directions.

Language and cultural barriers

Older persons may have a limited command of the dominant language of the country, or they may find their ability to understand instructions diminished by the stressful situation. The resulting failure in communication could easily be exacerbated by the presence of authority figures, such as police officers, who may increase the apprehension and confusion in the mind of older persons. Many older adults speak other languages, and there is a critical need to be sensitive to language and cultural differences. Older persons in this category may need special assistance in applying for disaster assistance.

Mobility impairment or limitation

Older persons may not have the ability to use automobiles or have access to private or public transportation. This may limit their ability to reach the disaster assistance centers, obtain goods or water, or relocate when necessary. Older persons may also have physical impairments which limit mobility.

Charity stigma

Many older persons are reluctant to accept not use services that have the connotation of being "charity." Older persons often have to be convinced that disaster services are available as a government service. Older persons need to know that their receipt of assistance will not keep another person who is worse-off from receiving help.

■■■ GROUP WORK/EXERCISES

Write a post-disaster script and role-play the following:

- A retired couple—wife 62 years old and husband 67 years old-who lose their home and go to a shelter
- A widow, 68 years old, whose house gets damaged
- A single man, 70 years of age, who moved in with his son, daughter-in-law, and 3 kids after his house was flooded.

Choose one vignette and develop the appropriate interventions.

PERSONS WITH MENTAL ILLNESS

■■■ **CONTENT SUMMARY**

Historical changes in the care of the people with mental illness and retardation and homeless persons living in the community have resulted in at-risk populations needing special help after a disaster. Although the number of such individuals housed in shelters or in damaged dwellings may be small in comparison to the total population, each case may need skillful handling and different approaches.

Although it is difficult to identify a general set of characteristics of survivors with mental problems, some generalities apply. Most of these survivors will need additional help beyond crisis intervention, but during the first chaotic days following a disaster it is important to ask several questions in order to assist mental health workers and clarify some guidelines for action. The following questions will help workers focus on the important points.

■ **HOW TO IDENTIFY THE MENTALLY ILL?**

Individuals suffering from a diverse variety of mental illnesses will exhibit differing reactions to the many stressors following a disaster. In a post-disaster situation, these individuals will fall into three major categories:

- **Individuals living in hospitals in damaged or physically inaccessible areas**: Problems in their daily living arrangements will have been disrupted by interference with the availability of electricity, water, food, medical care, and nursing staff.
- **Individuals living in group homes**: These individuals may be affected by loss of their homes, alteration of their surroundings, or limited access to medication. The loss of a familiar setting may increase the acuteness of their emotional reactions, which may, in turn, be manifested as symptomatology.
- **Individuals living with their own or foster families**: These individuals also may have increased symptoms due to factors similar to those for individuals living in group homes.

If individuals are accompanied by a familiar adult helper (a parent, for example), it may not be difficult to ascertain the diagnosis and the medication needed. This is not the case if the individual is discovered alone; in such cases, the signs of disturbance in cognition, disorientation, and communication problems (severe difficulty in explaining who he/she is and what has happened) will make it clear that this is an individual who needs special attention. Individuals who cannot follow simple, life-preserving instructions will need individual monitoring. However, during a disaster, it is always necessary to rule out any undiagnosed head injuries that might cause similar symptoms.

■ HOW TO DIFFERENTIATE BETWEEN THOSE SUFFERING FROM ACUTE STRESS AND THOSE WHO ARE MENTALLY ILL?

Individuals who manifest behavior that appears inappropriate for the situation should be given a rapid assessment to differentiate between individuals suffering from acute stress and those with mental illness according to whether they exhibit the following conditions:

• intense stress-reaction
• acute psychotic reaction
• effect of head injuries
• disorganization of functions in a mentally retarded individual

These four conditions are accompanied by several signs that differentiate them.

Stress reactions are manifested by (1) changes in cognition-orientation, memory, thinking, and difficulty in decision-making and (2) changes in emotions, lability, blunting, flatness. There is no break with reality awareness or loss of self-identify. The person behaves within social conventions and relates in a passive way during the acute stage.

Acute psychotic reactions have three severe manifestations which can be classified as expressions of anxiety, affective, and thinking behaviors. In general, it has been reported that diagnosed psychiatric patients behave in a subdued, calmer way than usual when they are faced with emergency situations. Some individuals may have a psychotic break if they suffer severe and prolonged trauma. Their behavior might range from apathetic, depressed, bizarre thinking, and difficulty in understanding the routine of the shelter/hospital to hyperactive, manic, unrealistic, and difficult to control.

The signs and symptoms of the **effect of head injuries** can mimic the characteristics of many psychiatric disorders, but a careful neurological exam may reveal localized signs of trauma. This diagnosis should be ruled out whenever a severe, acute clinical picture that indicating mental disorganization emerges.

Mentally retarded individuals may manifest disorganized and disoriented behavior due to the sudden changes in their routines. Their expressions of this new experience may include anxiety and infantile clinging behavior, which can be alleviated by simple instructions, support, and guidance. These individuals will manifest more infantile behaviors and have simple and concrete speech, as well as slowness in understanding instructions or suggestions.

■ HOW TO ASSIST THE MENTALLY ILL?

A number of individuals with mental illness are dependent on psychotherapeutic medications, and obtaining information about their regimen should be a priority. This should be followed by an attempt to structure their schedules and remove the patients from intense stimuli situations whenever possible. Using other survivors to assist in basic daily living activities may also be beneficial.

■ WHAT ARE SOME COMMON MEDICATION REGIMENS OF PERSONS WITH MENTAL ILLNESS?

Psychotropic medication is prescribed for different types of mental disorders. The three most common medications are antipsychotic drugs (for schizophrenic syndromes, for example) antidepressives (for minor and major depressive disorders), and lithium (for manic episodes of bipolar illness). Most patients are knowledgeable about their medication and would respond to inquiry in this regard.

■ WHAT ARE THE GUIDELINES FOR THE USE OF PSYCHOTROPIC MEDICATION WITH DISASTER SURVIVORS?

It is expected that the survivor will be assisted by a medical professional, but mental health workers should be aware of the following:

a) Basic medical precautions should be followed when prescribing medication to survivors. In general, the approach should be conservative in dealing with anxiety and psychophysiological reactions (headache, stomach ache, and sleeplessness), which are the primary manifestations during the first few days. Though survivors may wish to short circuit these very uncomfortable emotions, workers should consider first trying reassurance and counseling, with attention to the individual's living conditions, to determine whether the anxiety ameliorates without medication. If this does not happen, and psychological efforts are ineffective or the anxiety is overwhelming, then the worker should refer these survivors to a clinic.

b) Former mental patients (now living in the community)—for example, those individuals who have been diagnosed with schizophrenia or patients with dysthymic disorders (mania or depression)—will need continued monitoring of medication usage, as their judgment may become dysfunctional in the wake of a disaster.

WHAT TO DO ABOUT ANTISOCIAL BEHAVIOR PATTERNS IN EMERGENCY SITUATIONS?

Antisocial behavior is defined as the intrusive manner in which individuals clash with the norms of the community in which they live. Disaster survivors are suddenly and painfully thrown together in a desperate and unfamiliar setting. The behaviors that emerge as they try to cope and adapt might be defined by those in positions of authority as being "antisocial" because these individuals (1) break rules, (2) never seem to accept schedules, (3) refuse to take their turn dealing with helpers, and (4) in general are identified as "trouble-makers," who may also steal and lie. Diagnosing these behaviors and sorting out which are motivated by anxiety and which by personality disorders can challenge the skills of disaster workers.

Because diagnosis must be rapid during the emergency phase, it may be difficult to ascertain the motivating emotions driving antisocial behavior. The best approach is to increasingly set limits on disruptive actions.

Survivors who act out due to anxiety will experience relief if structure and support are provided. They will express mortification or guilt, and will verbalize some of their fears. In the case of aggressive, self-centered, and nonempathetic individuals, crisis workers need to use stronger measures, including segregation from the group, until more individual measures are available.

HOW TO DISTINGUISH ANTISOCIAL BEHAVIOR FROM A STRESS DISORDER?

Mr. B., a 34-year-old white male, was having difficulty sleeping. He complained about the discomfort and noise of the shelter and expressed irritation at all the rules that regimented his living activities. He was verbose, sarcastic, and angry. After an evaluation, it was decided that no medication would be prescribed but that he would be assigned a new sleeping area in the shelter. This change necessitated a rearrangement of bedding and Mr. B. did not like the new setting, either. He began to disobey the rules of group living and had problems in his unit, which prompted further investigation. He exhibited general annoyance, verbalized his dissatisfaction with rules, and boasted that he had "ways" of dealing with authority. In contrast to "stress-induced" behavior, his behavior was demanding, manipulative, and showed constant intrusion and lack of sensitivity to the rights of others, plus boasting of his "ability" to disobey authority.

An example of "increased limit-setting on disruptive actions" is provided by episodes in emergency wards where individuals begin to fight first verbally and then escalate to physical interchanges or actions against individuals that add misery to their living conditions. The first level of "limit-setting" is a personal discussion with the " survivor," which is followed by increasing control as the fighting escalates.

■ WHAT ARE THE SPECIAL NEEDS OF THE MENTALLY RETARDED?

Except for severely mentally retarded individuals, most retarded persons will not need special measures. Some may need assistance with instructions on how to manage in the shelter or obtain resources offered by agencies. Some careful explanation of what has happened and what plans have been made for the next few months may be of great relief to them. In cases where mental retardation is severe and accompanied by physical handicaps, it may be necessary to ask another survivor to assist in daily hygiene, feeding, and sleeping activities.

■ ARE THERE OTHER ILLNESS OR INJURIES THAT MASQUERADE AS RETARDATION?

There are many syndromes that are accompanied by symptoms of mental retardation. For example, an individual suffering from epilepsy may be taking an anticonvulsant, although such individuals may also have some degree of mental retardation.

■ HOW TO DEAL WITH EXTREME STRESS CAUSED BY THE EMERGENCY?

The information presented in previous chapters describes the interventions for addressing the emotional and cognitive reactions of survivors. Reactions to extreme stress are characterized by strong signs of fear, anxiety, disorganized speech, and inability to be consoled or quieted down. Most acute, severe reactions are short-lived when the survivor is surrounded by other individuals who are all in a similar situation and offer a role model for good coping. If the survivor has experienced physical injury, then his/her reactions will have to be evaluated in terms of pain, dependence, fear of abandonment, and central nervous system functional status as a reaction to trauma and/or medication.

■ WHAT RELOCATION FACTORS ARE LIKELY TO INCREASE/REDUCE STRESS?

One of the most painful conditions that survivors experience is a sensation of disorientation and lack of control over their lives. This experience is aggravated by further by the relocation that most survivors have to undergo. The process of preparing, supporting, and assisting survivors in all the location changes can intensify or ameliorate their discomfort. In their interactions with survivors, counselors should take into consideration the survivors' fear, anxiety and lack of knowledge about "the authorities" who are doing all the talking and making decisions and plans on their behalf. Any support or information that can be given to enhance survivors' sense of control over their choices, which in turn will moderate anxiety and elevate self-esteem, will be helpful. Keeping them closer to support systems, friends, clergy, and family will be beneficial to their recovery of psychological health. Communicating imminent changes to survivors will also be helpful.

■ HOW TO MOBILIZE SOCIAL SUPPORT SYSTEMS AFTER AN EMERGENCY?

During a disaster and its aftermath there is often an outpouring of interest and resources by individuals in the community. Hence, the problem with support systems is not quantity, but quality—i.e., finding the appropriate "fit" between the needs of the survivors (age, sex, culture, socioeconomic status, health, etc.) and the human interest and support available. The matching of assistance to survivors has to be organized in some effective manner, which may be flexible and simple, but with genuine and serious attention to motivation, consistency, and appropriateness.

There are many organized groups in different countries whose objectives are to assist individuals in crisis. Religious groups are also available to aid survivors who ask for assistance from persons with a specific religious affiliation.

A list of available groups could be identified by geographic region. Informational support groups (non-family), while generous and enthusiastic, may need some guidance and organization to assist survivors.

■ HOW TO LESSEN THE STRESS OF THE HOSPITAL SETTING AND RELOCATION?

Starting from the premise that the population housed in a hospital setting has been relocated and may face further relocation, it follows that some effects of the stressors will be manifested through psychophysiological reactions. How to lessen the stressor impact on these at-risk populations is the objective of disaster planners and workers. From the curriculum content presented in earlier chapters, two major types of emotional reaction emerge: (1) reactions to the event itself, including the rescue; and (2) reactions to hospital conditions. Not much can be done about the first source of stress, except to assist survivors in sharing their stories and venting some of their pent-up tensions. As for the second source of stress— living conditions in the hospital—some flexibility might be introduced with regard to the provision of information about their physical status and prognosis and guidance and support with schedules for medical intervention and present plans of care. Daily bulletins with clear information, coupled with methods to deal with rumors about what has happened to their neighborhood, are helpful.

A "problem-solving" hospital team can expedite simple requests or can educate survivors, explaining why some of their problems cannot be solved or attended to immediately. This type of communication can diminish expectations that could, if unchecked, culminate in further painful disappointments. Most survivors would prefer to be busy, active, and helpful, so any functions that can realistically be assigned to them will prove "moral- boosting."

Personnel trained to "absorb" painful, emotional, and angry expressions of distress, without reacting personally and becoming defensive or promising immediate solutions, may be one of the most valuable resources available to lower stress levels and mitigate survivors' reactions.

■ HOW TO COORDINATE HEALTH WITH MENTAL HEALTH?

Generally, mental health workers do not participate in the acute, emergency stage of disaster response, due to numerous organizational and budgetary constraints. This does not mean that government authorities in the affected region could not decide to allow public mental health professionals or appointed private systems to respond. Given the conditions in the acute phase, there is a need for pre-planning and a direct line of communication to mental health workers who are potentially available to participate in emergency operations. Once the decision to participate and the plan of action is in effect, mental health workers can assist in triage and debriefing operations, in consultation and case work-up, and in crisis intervention. To coordinate all these efforts smoothly, the administrative design should include mental health professionals in decision-making, logistics, scheduling, and setting functional priorities.

■ HOW CAN USE OF MENTAL HEALTH PROFESSIONALS IN THE INITIAL POST-DISASTER PERIOD ASSIST IN THE MEDICAL EMERGENCY INTERVENTION PROGRAM?

The mental health professional can bring expertise in crisis intervention techniques and medical knowledge of psychopharmacology to assist other members of the post-disaster health team. The scope of assistance will depend on the background and area of expertise, array of skills, and knowledge of the mental health team, whose members can range from psychiatrists specializing in crisis/emergency intervention, who would have the broadest base of experience for participating in the emergency response, to non-medical professionals who work in shelters and have little experience in crisis work. The assistance of mental health professionals has begun to enhance disaster emergency efforts because it brings a component of knowledge that is needed to deal with behavior patterns of not only the survivors but the helpers as well. The knowledge base of the mental health professionals working side by side with medical teams is continually increasing as more begin to practice "in the field." Mental health professionals should be considered members of every disaster triage health team. Their work, aimed at addressing psychophysiologic symptoms and reactions (affect, thinking, behavior) can be a valuable therapeutic addition to the medical emergency activities of a multidisciplinary post-disaster emergency effort.

PERSONS WITH HIV/AIDS

Individuals with HIV/AIDS present special challenges to the post-disaster worker. Due to the widespread myths and lack of knowledge about the transmission of HIV, survivors develop fear and anxiety when they find out that an individual who is HIV-positive is living, sleeping, or using the toilet facilities near them in a shelter. Mental health workers can help educate survivors and other crisis workers to reduce the fear of infection. Everyone involved in setting up post-disaster shelters needs to be able to plan to take care of patients with HIV infection, know the measures to prevent viral transmission, and be able to educate all workers to reduce unfounded fear of infection.

A grid like the one below, which shows four groups of people who may be present in a shelter, may be a helpful organizational tool for planning services for HIV-infected individuals.

Issue	HIV-infected Workers	HIV-infected Persons	HIV-negative Workers	HIV-infected Disaster Survivors
Medical	???	XXX	—	????
Social/sexual activity	—	???	—	???
Psychological problems/stress	XX	XXXXX	XX	XXX
Legal rights	X	XX	X	XX

The question marks signal that individuals who may not be identified as infected may pose a problem for shelter management in the "issue" area listed in the left column. The symbol "X" signifies that the issue must be considered when dealing with the care of an HIV-infected person in a shelter. As an example of how the grid might be used, if there is a strong suspicion that there may be an HIV-infected person in the shelter, the issue of how to deal with his/her social/sexual activity will have strong implications for prevention of HIV transmission, the individual's level of experienced stress, and his/her legal rights.

Some of the problems that need attention are:

• Reliance on volunteers in times of disaster necessarily results in a mix of values, attitudes, and cultural characteristics, as well as various levels of emergency preparedness among workers.

- Few volunteer shelter personnel are familiar with public health regulations and procedures for dealing with HIV-infected individuals in disaster situations.
- Training for shelter managers generally does not include content and skills relating to the mental health care of persons with HIV infection or of those living in close proximity to them.
- Experienced disaster workers are more comfortable with HIV-related information than new, inexperienced workers.
- In a disaster, there is a phenomenon of focusing on some problem, perhaps even a small one, which may provide some sense of control for disaster survivors.

■ TWELVE-POINT KNOWLEDGE BASE NEEDED BY WORKERS IN POST-DISASTER PROGRAMS

1. Recognition that individuals with HIV/AIDS are a new at-risk population in disaster assistance planning.
2. Identification of the unique needs of HIV-infected survivors, including medical, psychosocial, and legal needs.
3. Development within emergency agencies of clear lines of responsibility for the needs of individuals with HIV/AIDS in shelters, specialized housing, and hospitals.
4. Planning in a coordinated structure to link medical and government agencies to address the needs of survivors diagnosed with HIV/AIDS.
5. Incorporation in all training and emergency manuals of emergency care guidelines for the care of disaster survivors with HIV/AIDS.
6. Development of an inventory of existing and potential resources to respond to HIV/AIDS-related problems, including availability of health and mental health personnel; capabilities of the public health system, prison system, and mental health institutions; and preparedness of existing community-based organizations and networks, transportation and geographic location of shelters, etc.
7. Development of training materials about disaster management for incorporation in all community HIV/AIDS training programs.
8. Development of a "shelter-model" process to deal with the day-to-day problems of disaster survivors living with individuals who are HIV-infected or have AIDS.
9. Development of community emergency models for coordinating community-based HIV/AIDS services with government emergency response systems. Such models should focus on preplanning and prevention approaches to the care of HIV-infected disaster survivors
10. Awareness of the legal rights of individuals with HIV/AIDS in times of disaster in keeping with federal, state/provincial, and local laws concerning handicapped, HIV-infected, and at-risk individuals.

generally is booming in disaster areas. They will be surrounded by people who come from all over the country to work on the reconstruction. Alcohol and drug abuse is sometimes a problem among these people.

2. Females

Many female addicts are single mothers with small children. They are normally given priority for housing, usually in trailers, where they do not have to pay rent. These survivors also often receive public assistance or subsidies to cover the cost of food. Even though their situation appears to be stable, there may be nothing to eat in their homes and their children may not have suitable clothing to attend school because their mothers are spending the money on drugs and alcohol. There are many female addicts who are already in trouble with public child protective services because their babies tested positive for cocaine or other drugs at the time of birth. After the disaster, they may stop attending their mandatory treatment programs. They may request help in obtaining outpatient treatment that they are required to complete, but there may not be an outpatient treatment program available, or the available ones may not provide child care while the client is receiving services.

Addicted mothers may tend to physically abuse their children. This situation may be exacerbated by the traumatic experience of a disaster. Some females addicts make efforts toward getting a job, but due to their instability they are unable to keep their jobs.

C. Types of trauma found among survivors who are substance abusers

1. Loss of home.
  a) Not many "hard core" addicts are homeowners before a disaster. After a disaster, the alcohol-drug addiction problem tends to worsen. May addicts may spend a substantial amount of any money they receive from insurance companies or public assistance agencies on drugs and alcohol.
2. Loss of employment
  a) Addicts may lose their employment after a disaster due to the destruction of their workplace or lack of transportation. Their vehicles may also be destroyed. Loss of employment means less money, but for addicts this situation does not reduce their use of alcohol/drugs. On the contrary, the frustrating situation often contributes to increased substance abuse.
  b) Unemployed addicts need money to support their habit. For that reason, they may get involved in illegal activities, such as dealing drugs, robbery, and burglary.

The loss of their living quarters, combined with the fact that they are too distracted, confused, or sick to take the necessary steps to secure other housing, may impel them to settle in the remains of any domicile that remains standing after the disaster.

Loss of or separation from family members, some of whom may move to trailer parks or other parts of the city, adds to their loneliness.

If they move in with relatives, disparities in levels of acculturation between household members adds to the problem. This inconsistent family interaction becomes a major obstacle to counselors working with substance abuse cases. Incongruities in perceptions between different generations, in addition to the addict's deficient communication skills, make it very difficult to work on concepts such as co-dependency or create appropriate support systems.

Homelessness is another problem among survivors who are substance abusers. For diverse reasons, most of these survivors choose to live in makeshift camps, which makes follow-up almost impossible. Even if the counselor is able to locate them, they usually "disappear" again.

Yet another problem is unstable participation in the workforce. Work opportunities are not always available. In the case of the Hurricane Andrew disaster, this problem was compounded by "labor ripoffs." Many of these survivors reported at least one incident in which they were hired by a contractor who did not pay them.

■ DESCRIPTION OF EMOTIONAL STATUS

The most frequently recurring feeling found among this population after the Hurricane Andrew disaster was the stress produced by occupational and financial concerns (i.e., the frustration produced by their inability to get a job, lack of proper skills, and their legal and or "survivor" status). Another recurring feeling reported by many substance abusers was a strong feeling of inadequacy, usually associated with insufficient income to support their families.

Resignation and helplessness was commonly found, especially among survivors who had unresolved marital problems, and/or acculturation problems between family members.

Fear was also found among most survivors who were substance abusers. This feeling was usually manifested as displaced anger and distorted perceptions that led to maladaptive behaviors and reactions to severe stress.

Although some signs of anxiety were visible among minority population, in general, survivors who had been directly exposed to war and its consequences appeared more severely traumatized. Apparently, disasters trigger recurrent emotions and behaviors associated with destruction and chaos (i.e. intrusive thoughts of war-related deaths of family members or friends).

■ METHODS FOR IDENTIFYING SURVIVORS WHO ARE SUBSTANCE ABUSERS

Mental health teams should conduct door-to-door outreach assessments. All team members should participate in this operation. One question that should be asked in all households is whether there is a problem of substance abuse. If the interviewed family member admits to a drug/alcohol problem in the family, the team member conducting the assessment interview should refer the family to a substance abuse specialist.

Since not many people readily admit such a problem, the members of the team should be trained to recognize the signs of substance abuse in the family, such as beer cans outside, a messy house, lack of food, neglected children, smells, and, especially, hesitation in answering questions. They should be instructed that if they suspect a substance abuse problem, they should make a referral. The technique is to win the survivor's trust by asking unrelated questions and engaging the person in conversation. Sooner or later, in most cases, the survivor will open up and admitted to a drug/alcohol problem.

■ ASCERTAINING SURVIVORS' STATUS AND NEEDS

Once a survivor has admitted to having a drug/alcohol problem and agreed to receive help, the counselor should refer and assist him/her in finding an assessment and treatment agency.

Unless survivors readily acknowledge a substance abuse problem for which they want assistance, the counselor's intervention should take the form of empathic concern about their present circumstances and provision of any material assistance possible over a period of time until trust is established. Then the counselor can broach the subject of treatment, discussing options to fit their circumstances. If survivors are resistant, the counselor should let some time pass, during which their situation often becomes worse. The counselor can then approach them again, always making sure that they know how to reach help if they want it.

The objectives are to get substance abusers into treatment if possible or to plant the idea of getting treatment later if it is not possible to do so immediately in the disaster situation. An attempt should also be made to link the substance abuser's family members to sources of assistance.

1. When a survivor will not admit to having a problem with drugs/alcohol, the counselor should look for an excuse to come back to the house and try to get acquainted further with the survivor, establish rapport, and earn the survivor's confidence. The counselor should engage the survivor in a general, social conversation.
2. If the family is willing to cooperate, the family intervention approach can be used to assist in referral of the survivor for treatment. When possible, as many family members or significant others as possible can arrange a meeting with the survivor, and the counselor can proceed with the referral. This method, followed by arrangement with a treatment facility to receive the survivor, has proved effective.
3. Some survivors suffer from both drug addiction and mental health problems. They should be referred to a mental health facility.

▰▰▰ TEACHING RESOURCES

▰ GROUP WORK/EXERCISES

Exercise 1: Family post-disaster response

Videotape: *Hurricane Blues* (Available from Emergency Services and Disaster Relief Branch, Center for Mental Health Services, Washington, D.C., United States), or a similar video.

1. The instructor divides the students into groups, and assigns each group to list one of the following after viewing the video:
  • Emotional expressions
  • Behavior of family members
  • Dynamic interaction:
    a) Between children
    b) Between adults
    c) Between children and adults
2. As a group, the students list the objectives of intervention to assist the family.
3. Each student picks one objective and role-plays the technique of intervention.

Note: The instructor should stop the tape before the counselor presentation portion and proceed with the exercise. After the exercise is completed, play the counselor presentation portion and discuss.

Exercise 2

Videotape: *Children and Disaster* (available from Emergency Services and Disaster Relief Branch, Center for Mental Health Services, Washington, D.C., United States), or a similar video.

The instructor shows the videotape and the entire group discusses the presentation and intervention techniques.

Exercise 3

The instructor asks the students to list the problems posed by the subpopulation of survivors with mental illness and HIV/AIDS.

Exercise 4

The instructor asks the students to write a script and act out several episodes of situations faced by elderly survivors.

DISASTER WORKERS

■■■ INTRODUCTION TO ASSISTING WORKERS AND SECONDARY VICTIMS OF DISASTERS

Exposure to traumatic stress among rescue and post-disaster workers participating in emergency operations may lead to the development of cumulative stress reactions, including post-traumatic stress disorder (PTSD), depression, and signs of "burn-out." Systematic assistance, providing the opportunity to receive help and specific modalities of intervention known as "defusing" and "debriefing," will help support these workers and reduce the impact of disaster effects. The trainer will present the description of the different techniques and formats.

Workers in all aspects of disaster relief—whether emergency services, shelters or clothing/food services operated by nongovernmental organizations, governmental rehabilitation and reclamation services, or human service workers—expose themselves to unprecedented personal demands in their desire to help meet the needs of survivors. For many, the disaster takes precedence over all other responsibilities and activities, and the workers devote all their time to disaster-created tasks, at least in the immediate post-impact period. They should be trained to expect "burn-out," so that they may recognize the signs, not only in themselves but also in their fellow workers. All levels of administration and management personnel should also be alert to burn-out so that they can assist workers in a disaster. As some order returns, many of the workers return to their regular jobs, but at the same time attempt to continue with their disaster work. As mentioned previously, the result of the overwork is the burn-out syndrome, a state of exhaustion, irritability, and fatigue which creeps up on the individual unrecognized and undetected, markedly decreasing his/her effectiveness and capability.

The best way to forestall the burn-out syndrome is to expect it, be alert to its early signs, and actively seek to relieve stress. Four primary areas of symptomatology have been identified.

■ SYMPTOMS

Thinking

Mental confusion, slowness of thought, inability to make judgments and decisions, loss of ability to conceptualize alternatives or to prioritize tasks, loss of objectivity in evaluating own functioning, etc.

Psychological

Depression, irritability, anxiety, hyperexcitability, excessive rage reactions, loss of control, etc.

Somatic

Physical exhaustion, loss of energy, gastrointestinal distress, appetite disturbances, hypochondria, sleep disorders, tremors, etc.

Behavioral

Hyperactivity, excessive fatigue, impulsiveness, inability to express oneself verbally or in writing, etc.

Disasters bring together emergency service workers from diverse backgrounds. Some arrive immediately with clear responsibility and government-mandated priority assignments. Others arrive with different levels of previous experience and skills and different assigned post-disaster jobs. All emergency workers—for example, "first responder" teams—attempt to be helpful and proceed to rescue the wounded, gather the dead, and use triage methods to determine the priority of intervention. They work long hours with little thought to food or sleep. This group of workers represents a challenge for planning and operationalizing a program of post-disaster intervention. Programs geared toward the different teams that work with survivors for long periods of time should be put in place to monitor and prevent stress reactions.

The importance of contemporary approaches to identify, understand, and assist post-disaster workers suffering from stress reactions has been documented. Jeffrey Mitchell and colleagues have produced training materials outlining the history of critical incident stress and common reactions and symptoms experienced by emergency workers (see Reading List).

The same conceptual "building-blocks" of knowledge presented in the basic mental health component of this book provide guidelines for assisting workers in the daily performance of their painful jobs. Workers are also under severe stress—especially those who are both survivors and rescue workers—due to time pressures and job commitments.

Each type of post-disaster worker works within different organizations that interrelate within the common goal of disaster assistance. Multiple individuals are recruited to a site to help, with little opportunity to identify or work out a good fit between worker and assignment. This situation generally produces role conflict, ambiguity, and discomfort. Workers generally have multiple functions. They often attend to diverse, and at times, conflicting, needs of survivors. The mental health worker should focus on the emotional impact of these stressors on disaster workers, as well as their reactions, behavior, and feelings, as a guide for selecting the best methods of helping them do their jobs. These reactions can range from good coping and growth to pathological and chronic sequelae that leave a dysfunctional individual and persist for months after the worker has returned to his/her home and previous job. Multiple variables interact at a given historical moment in the life of the worker, which accounts for such widely divergent outcomes.

An important concept that encompasses many aspects of this occupational stress has been labeled "burn-out," which is characterized by mental and emotional exhaustion with physiological manifestations—sleep disturbances, appetite problems, increased irritability—all of which interferes with work. The phenomenon of burn-out has many sources, but an obvious major one is that most disaster workers are not taught or assisted during the relief operation to look for, identify, and address their own physical and emotional needs. They do not acknowledge that their needs are normal in these very abnormal situations and that, unless they meet their needs continuously, they will not be able to function in a supportive, consistent, and sensitive manner to help survivors.

Various approaches are available to disaster trainers, planners, and program directors to prevent burn-out and assist workers as they function in disasters. These methods help workers acquire techniques and skills for coping with stress. The importance of exercise, diet, relaxation, and recreation is now recognized in employment conditions and should be emphasized in ongoing training activities for workers.

Mental health crisis counselors who are employed to assist survivors are also now available to assist other workers in debriefing meetings and critical incident stress debriefing sessions.

■ DEBRIEFING

Debriefing focuses on the cognitive and emotional reactions of workers who are trying to cope with novel internal sensations that accumulate from their work experiences. Debriefing interventions are done in small groups, with specific objectives and confidentiality boundaries. The structure of the debriefing includes the following sequence of processes:

- Description of the workers' activities in interacting with survivors: Participants share and reconstruct scenarios—visual, auditory, and olfactory.
- Identification and recognition of paradoxical or unusual emotional reactions of workers: This reduces misconceptions, corrects misinformation, and identifies methods of stress reduction.
- Recognition of ambivalent feelings in some situations and their significance for the worker.
- Linkage of feelings to physiological manifestations: Workers are helped to see the linkage between some of their feelings and the disturbance of sleep, appetite, impulse control, and irritability that they may experience following a stressful assignment.
- The mental health worker summarizes the discussion, answers questions, and reinforces the message that emergency workers' responses are normal reactions to abnormal situations. This approach also provides an opportunity to support and reinforce coping efforts.

A critical incident session is generally conducted with individuals who have participated in extremely traumatic situations and are experiencing signs of psychophysiological stress that they are finding it difficult to cope with and overcome. A very important condition of such sessions is that they should be completely confidential and nonjudgmental.

■ CRITICAL INCIDENT RESPONSE

An incident occurs: it is sudden, random, and stressful. It affects not only the survivor, but the workers as well. The incident can shatter their sense of safety and well-being and temporarily destroy their ability to function normally.

This reaction is called a "critical incident response." Although individuals will react with differing degrees of intensity and recover at varying rates, most individuals will go through some form of critical incident response, which may involve an alteration between two states: numbness and hyperarousal, or being in control and powerlessness.

The objective of the Critical Incident Stress Debriefing (CISD) is to offer catharsis and education. The CISD should be offered within the first few days following the incident. The participants will be encouraged to share their feelings and reactions so that they can be helped to understand what has happened, put it into context, and learn the normal reactions expected in the specific situation.

■ DEFUSING

This process allows workers to vent or "blow off steam" in an informal, unstructured setting that can be organized following a day's work. At these meetings, guidance, advice, and information can be exchanged. If needed, these meetings can be followed by a formal, planned CISD or debriefing meeting.

The following pages are ready for use as transparencies, slides, or handouts.

BURN-OUT IN WORKERS

Definition
A state of mild, moderate, or severe exhaustion, irritability, and fatigue which markedly decrease an individual's effectiveness.

Coping Process
Process through which the worker tolerates or decreases the negative effects of an experience or masters a threatening situation.

Functions and Role Shift: Mental Health Worker to Disaster Worker

- Common knowledge base
- Different and novel variety of functions
- New attitudes — co-professional
- Rhythm and timing — crisis contingencies
- Evolution in expectations and attitudes of non-mental-health disaster assistance workers
- Participatory and collaborative consultation

BASIC CONCEPTUAL FRAMEWORK
BIO-PSYCHO-SOCIAL ORGANISM

Support Systems (Mediators — Regulators)

Assistance (at every level) to the individual in the aftermath of disaster - person-to-person exchange.

- Provide support for identification

- Exchange of helpful information

- Opportunity to share coping techniques

- Support increased sense of worth

- Reinforcement for change and maintenance of effort (feedback on performance)

- Provide concrete aid and serve as counselors

- Problem-solving options and prioritization of solutions

- Supporting activity, supporting empowerment in the face of adverse conditions

CONDITIONS PRESENT IN OCCUPATIONAL STRESS

- Time pressures

- Work overload

- Minimal positive reinforcement

- High probability of conflict

- Prolonged expenditure of energy and attention to survivors

- Coincidental incidents of crisis involving several survivors at the same time

- Personal crisis in the life of the post-disaster worker

BURN-OUT AS A PSYCHOPHYSIOLOGIC PROCESS AND STRATEGIES FOR MANAGING DISTRESS

PREVENTION THROUGH MANAGEMENT

1. Learn to recognize the stresses inherent in high-risk work and develop preventive strategies for mitigating those stresses.

2. Learn to recognize and assess signs and symptoms of stress when they occur and develop approaches and goals for managing such stress (coping and use of support systems).

3. Become aware that prevention and treatment strategies can potentially decrease or eliminate negative effects of stress and its consequences:

   Decline in job performance

   Burn-out

   High turnover rate

   Health problems

   Family problems for workers

4. Support system and resources available to workers for dealing with crisis situations — debriefing, counseling, education — are preventive methods for avoiding burn-out.

BARRIERS TO THE USE OF PREVENTIVE METHODS TO DIMINISH STRAIN AND BURN-OUT

1. High professional standards and high self-expectations among workers influence appraisal of a situation

2. Reluctance or discomfort in discussing feelings, especially those that might connote weakness and reflect doubt about one's performance (self-appraisal)

3. Need to deny or suppress feelings during difficult situations in order to function: discomfort in acknowledging and discussing those feelings when they emerge and produce strain

4. Concern that acknowledging psychological assistance will reflect negatively on job performance evaluations, opportunities for promotion (values, belief systems)

5. Workers may have difficulties in judging their own reactions and performance when they are overwhelmed and distressed

6. Shame and guilt over the contrast between the worker's personal situations and that of survivors

BUFFERS TO MITIGATE BURN-OUT

1. Extensive training protects from physical and emotional strain

2. Available repertoire of coping strategies

3. Realistic self-expectations and role boundaries

4. Control of over-identification with survivors

5. Awareness of fantasies of "omnipotence"

6. Minimal role confusion

7. Modification of identified negative coping

8. Practice of positive coping

9. Comfort in using support system and helpful supervision

CHARACTERISTICS OF CRITICAL INCIDENTS & PSYCHOLOGICAL RESULTS

Support Guidelines for Workers

1. Workers should have a plan for communicating with and locating their families.

2. Workers should be aware of conditions in the field before reporting to their work sites.

3. Workers should obtain necessary supplies, including information on disaster worker stress management and self-care.

4. Workers should ascertain chain of command and supervision from operations center to field staff.

5. Teams should establish roles and responsibilities.

6. Workers should develop team coordination with other community resources, e.g., Red Cross, disaster health and mental health services.

7. Workers should watch for signs of stress among their colleagues and receive continuing training, guidance, and supervision.

CRITICAL SITUATION STRESS DEBRIEFING PROCESS

1. High-risk workers are potentially vulnerable to physical and psychological responses to human suffering, crisis situations, and death.

2. Effective methods exist to help workers cope with what they are experiencing in dealing with overwhelming crisis situations.

3. A "critical incident" can be defined as one that generates unusually strong feelings in the worker and can become a memory that triggers previous emotional reactions.

4. Debriefing is a new form of supervision and crisis resolution for high-risk workers involved in jobs entailing conditions of daily stress.

5. This process helps alleviate the worker's stress responses following tragic situations in dealing with crisis survivors. It also helps prevent delayed stress reactions which may appear weeks later.

VICTIMS AND HELPERS

Helpers as Hidden Victims

	MOTIVATION		REPONSE	OUTCOME
"HELPERS"		Altruistic Response (positive Curiosity)	Coping by:	Positive:
	Personal Motivation		Active Doing Mastery Review	Good Helping, Positive Life Experience
	Perceptions of Disaster			
	Perception of Helping		Supportive Relationships	Negative:
	Past Experience		Emotional Release	Poor Helping, Negative Life Experience
	Personality Factors			
				Psychological Disorder
"VICTIMS"	Death Encounter	Anguish of Others	Role Stresses	
	Loss and Other Stresses			

GOALS OF DEBRIEFING*

1. Ensure that the participant's basic needs are met.

2. Have the participants share, verbally reconstruct, and ventilate the most acute, intense emotions and memories of the disaster.

3. Help the participants to explore the symbolic meaning of the event.

4. Nurture reassurance about the "normality" of the participants' reactions and reduce feelings of uniqueness.

5. Facilitate group support and enhance peer social supports.

6. Reduce misconceptions and correct misinformation about events and about "normal" and "abnormal" stress reactions.

7. Encourage, teach, and reinforce coping efforts.

8. Assist group in discussing methods for reducing tension and anxiety.

9. Help facilitate the return to routine pre-incident functioning and encourage group assistance.

10. Screen and refer "high-risk" participants for professional assistance.

11. Emphasize that one purpose of debriefing is to reconstruct what really happened so that others may benefit from the lessons learned.

* Based on the publications by JT Mitchell et al. (see Reading List).

POST TRAUMA STRESS DEBRIEFINGS

Post trauma recovery trainings are most effective when they occur 2 to 5 days after the incident.

Debriefings should be mandatory for all personnel involved in the incident and should follow this format:

A. Introduction to Debriefing

To begin the debriefing, any necessary introductions are made. The ground rules, including confidentiality, are discussed and the agenda is presented.

B. Telling the Story

Each debriefing participant describes his/her experiences and feelings during the critical incident.

C. Sharing Responses and Reactions

Each debriefing participant describes his/her post-trauma responses.

D. Understanding the Responses and Reactions

Information concerning post-trauma stress is presented, including the normal results of exposure to post-trauma stress and expectations for recovery.

E. "Contracting" for Recovery

Each participant develops a plan for recovery that will assist in the management of post-trauma stress and reduce the possibility of long-term post-traumatic stress.

F. Closing

The debriefing is terminated and contact is made with participants.

Small group debriefings include a follow-up session three to four weeks after the initial session.

(This debriefing process is a modification of the Post-shooting Debriefing developed by the U.S. Federal Bureau of Investigation and Jeff Mitchell's Critical Incident Stress Debriefing.)

SMALL GROUP DEBRIEFING

No more than 15 participants

Primary goal: Management of post-trauma consequences and assessment by debriefers

- All participants discuss their experiences for the purpose of sharing details and the benefits of venting their feelings.

- All participants report their post-trauma consequences.

- Support provided to each participant from other group members, department, and debriefers.

- Discussion of event by each participant.

- Understanding by listening to other participants and information provided concerning the normalcy of post-trauma responses.

CRITICAL INCIDENT DEBRIEFING

- Participants are selected for further services based on facilitators' assessment of condition and severity of post-trauma consequences.

- Duration of at least two to three hours; difficult to control time.

- Follow-up must occur.

- Assessment by debriefing facilitators of all participants and determination of the need for further services. Referrals to more intense services as required.

- Follow-up in a few weeks to observe any development of long-term reactions and provision of another assessment.

POST-TRAUMA STRESS DEBRIEFING

Suggested Post-trauma "Do's and Don'ts"

Depending on the traumatic incident and post-trauma consequences, these are examples of coping skills for debriefing participants.

DO	DON'T
Get ample rest	Drink alcohol excessively
Maintain a good diet and exercise	Use legal or illegal substances to numb feelings.
Take time for leisure activities	Withdraw from significant others
Structure your life as much as possible but recognize you may not always follow through	Stay away from work
Find and talk to supportive peers and/or family members about the incident	Reduce amount of leisure activities
Learn about post-trauma stress	Have unrealistic expectations for the success of post-disaster counseling recovery
Spend time with family and friends	Look for easy answers to help survivors
Expect the incident to produce strong emotions	Make major life changes or decisions at this time
Get extra help from a post-trauma reaction specialist, clergy person, supervisor	Be too hard on yourself or others- reflect on issues and try to put them into perspective

TRAUMATIC INCIDENT STRESS DEBRIEFING ACTION PLAN

EXERCISE, RELAXATION, SPIRITUAL ACTIVITIES, REST

Activities to help my recovery
(in the immediate future and the long term):

To take care of myself I will. . .
(Plan and carry out a coping activity)

Today:

This Week:

This Month:

■ GROUP WORK/EXERCISES

• Ask each member of the group to present a difficult event that has occurred in his/her life.
• Obtain a video that shows the techniques of debriefing. React to the process; analyze the steps.
• List the "do's" and "don'ts" when assisting a disaster worker using "critical incident debriefing."
• Role-play a "defusing" session with a small subgroup of students and have the rest of the students observe and analyze the procedures used. ■

READING LIST

American Academy of Pediatrics Work Group on Disasters. *Psychosocial issues for children for children and families in disasters.* Washington, D.C.: U.S. Department of Health and Human Services; 1995. (DHHS Publication No. (SMA) 95-3022).

Armstrong K et al. Multiple stressor debriefing and the American Red Cross: The East Bay Hills fire experience. *Social Work* 1995;40(1): 83-90.

Bell J. Traumatic event debriefing: service delivery designs and role of social work. *Social Work* 1995; 40(1): 36-43.

Bergman KH, Queen TR. Critical incident stress: Parts I and II. *Fire Command* 1986: 18-20, 52-56.

Boyd Webb N (ed.). *Helping bereaved children.* New York: The Guilford Press; 1993.

Burke JD, Borus JF, Burns BJ et al. Some factors in the emotional reaction of children to disaster. *American Journal of Psychiatry* 1982;139:1010-1014.

Center for Mental Health Services. *Psychosocial issues for older adults in disasters.* Rockville, Maryland: CMHS; 1999. (DHHS Publication No. ESDRB SMA 99-3323).

Cohen R, Culp C, Genser S. *Human problems in major disasters: a training curriculum for emergency medical personnel.* Washington, D.C.; Government Printing Office; 1987. (DHHS Publication No. (ADM) 87-1505).

Cohen RE. Intervention program for children. In: Lystad M (ed.). *Mental health for mass emergencies: theory and practice.* New York: Brunner/Mazel; 1988: pp. 262-283.

Cohen RE, Poulshock S. The elderly in the aftermath of a disaster. *Gerontologist* 1975;15:357-361.

Duckworth DH. Psychological problems arising from disaster work. *Stress Medicine* 1986;2:315-323.

Dyregov A. Caring for helpers in disaster situations: psychological debriefing. *Disaster Management* 1989; 2: 25-30.

Eth S. *Responding to disaster: a guide for mental health professionals, clinical response to traumatized children.* Washington, DC: American Psychiatric Press, Inc.; 1992: pp. 101-123.

Faber NIL, Gorton N. *Manual for child health workers in major disaster.* Rockville, Maryland: National Institute of Mental Health; 1986. (DHHS Publication No. (ADM) 86-1070).

Hartsough DM, Myers DG. *Disaster work and mental health: prevention and control of stress among workers.* Rockville, Maryland: National Institute of Mental Health; 1985. (DHHS Pub No (ADM) 85-1422).

Kenardy JA, Webster RA, Lewing TJ, Carr VJ, Hazell PL, Carter GL. Stress debriefing and patterns of recovery following a natural disaster. *Journal of Traumatic Stress* 1996; 9:37-49.

Kilinanek T, Drabek T. Assessing long-term impacts of a natural disaster: a focus on the elderly. *The Gerontologist* 1979;19(6):555-566.

Klingman A, Koenigsfeld E, Markman D. Art activity with children following disaster. *Arts Psychotherapy* 1987;14:153-166.

Krause N. Exploring the impact of a natural disaster on the health and psychological well-being of older adults. *Journal of Human Stress* 1987;13(2): 61-69.

Lima B et al. Disaster severity and emotional disturbance: implications for primary mental health care in developing countries. *Acta Psychiatr* 1989;79:74-82.

McFarlane AC. Post-traumatic phenomena in a longitudinal study of children following a natural disaster. *Journal of the American Academy of Child and Adolescent Psychiatry* 1987;26:764-769.

Mitchell JT. Helping the helper. In: Lystad M (ed.).: *Role stressors and supports for emergency workers.* Washington, D.C.: Government Printing Office; 1984: pp. 105-118. (DHHS Publication No. (ADM) 85-1908).

Mitchell JT. Too much help too fast. *Life Net* 1995; *5:3-4.*

Mitchell JT. When disaster strikes: the critical incident stress debriefing. *Journal of Emergency Medical Services* 1983;8: 36-39.

Mitchell M, Bray G. *Emergency services stress: guidelines for preserving the health and careers of emergency services personnel.* Englewood Cliffs, New Jersey: Prentice Hall; 1990.

National Institute of Mental Health. *Preventive and control of stress among workers: a pamphlet for workers.* Rockville, Maryland: NIMH; 1987. (DHHS Publication No. (ADM) 87-1496).

National Institute of Mental Health. *Responding to the needs of people with serious and persistent mental illness in times of major disaster.* Rockville, Maryland: NIMH; 1996. (DHHS Pub. No. (ADM) 96-3077).

Phifer JF, Kaniasty KZ, Norris FH. The impact of natural disaster on the health of older adults: a multiwave prospective study. *Journal of Health and Social Behavior* 1988;29:65-78.

Shalev AY. Debriefing following traumatic exposure. In: Ursano RJ, McCaughey BC, Fullerton CS (eds.). *Individual and community responses to trauma and disaster: the structure of human chaos.* Cambridge: Cambridge University Press; 1996: pp. 201-219.

Talbot A. The importance of parallel process in debriefing crisis counsellors. *Journal of Traumatic Stress* 1990;3: 265-278.

The following publications can be obtained from the U.S. Department of Health and Human Services, Center for Mental Health Services, Emergency and Disaster Relief Branch, Rockville, Maryland 20857 USA.

Disaster Work and Mental Health: Prevention and Control of Stress Among Workers, 1985 (reprinted 1987).

Manual for Child Health Workers in Major Disasters, 1981 (reprinted 1986)

Prevention and Control of Stress Among Emergency Workers: A Pamphlet for Team Managers, 1987 (reprinted 1988, 1990).

Psychological Issues for Children and Families in Disasters: A Guide for the Primary Care Physician, 1995.

Psychosocial Issues for Older Adults in Disasters, 1999.

Responding to the Needs of People with Serious and Persistent Mental Illness in Times of Major Disaster, 1996.

Role Stressors and Supports for Emergency Workers, 1985 (reprinted 1990).

Training Manual for Human Service Workers in Major Disasters, 1978 (reprinted 1983, 1986, 1990).

This work has been published by
Pan American Health Organization
in coedition with
Editorial El Manual Moderno, S.A. de C.V.,
and was printed in august 25th, 2000
in Programas Educativos, S.A. de C.V.,
Calz. Chabacano No. 65, Local A,
Col. Asturias, 06850
A certified company by
Instituto Mexicano de Normalización y Certificación A.C.,
under the norm ISO-9002:1994/NMX-CC-004:1995
with register number RSC-048
Mexico, D.F.

1st. edition, 2000

●